ACNE

Just Another Four-Letter Word

by

Aarti Patel, N.D.

For my heroes, Lukas and Alisa

TABLE OF CONTENTS

PART 1
ACNE'S BAD WORDS

CHAPTER 1
Meet the Real Face of Acne

———•———

Every person who deals with acne knows something important about this skin condition that no one ever talks about. The mind and body are both involved. We want acne to be just a physical symptom so badly, but anyone who's had chronic persistent breakouts knows that we not only "have acne," we also live it and *think* about it all the time. First thing in the morning. Before bedtime. Out in social situations, and even when we're interacting with those we know well at home. All of a sudden, acne is not a simple physical symptom. It's a word that carries a lot of weight in our lives. It becomes our way of life. Our full-time job then becomes finding a fix for acne.

It's a desperate mission, and I know this from experience. I'm a naturopathic doctor now who works with patients dealing with acne and other chronic health issues. Once upon a time though, I was a teenager and eventually an adult who was always trying to run from the red and irritated bumps on my face. Wherever I turned, there they were.

When I was a year into college and couldn't take it anymore, I asked my mom to take me to the dermatologist. A specific combination of pharmaceutical treatments helped out my situation, and the prescribed topical medication cleared up my acne during my late teens and early twenties. This was a good time for my skin, but the medicine rose in cost each year and I was also starting to wonder: Where did the acne go? It may seem a strange thought from someone who was so desperate to kick acne's butt, but I felt suspicious about chemicals that could immediately wipe away my body's symptoms. I had always been interested in health, and this magical disappearing act of acne didn't seem healthy or natural.

Once insurance stopped covering the prescriptions and I started living life without them, I was met with a horrifying sight in the mirror. Underneath the surface, my skin had retaliated and the acne was worse than ever. Rather than clustering around my cheeks with an occasional bump on my chin, the new colonies of acne set up their homes everywhere. Even on my forehead. I was in my mid-twenties at the time, and it was not a period of my life when I wanted to deal with acne again. I missed my "perfect" skin, the kind I had enjoyed before I hit my teenage years. The kind that pharmaceutical drugs had made superficially possible.

My new life's purpose became fixing my skin. Like many people dealing with acne, I tried drugstore acne products, natural treatments, and homemade concoctions. I stopped eating foods that allegedly made acne worse, and I scoured the web for highly reviewed skin care lines. Often when you're determined to solve a problem, your options should become clearer, but the more I searched, the more hopeless I felt. "I'm doing all the right things," I thought, "but it's not making any difference!" In fact, my skin was getting worse over time as my frustration grew.

Still, I kept on researching about acne, day after day. Eventually I turned toward a career in naturopathic medicine because I knew acne was affecting my health on more than just a superficial level. I wanted to find out what was going on at the root of my symptoms, and one day I hoped to help other people who were going through what I was going through. But first I had to help myself. The question was: What was I really going through? What does anyone go through when acne takes hold of their life?

We are led to believe that the biggest challenges we're facing involve things like hormones, clogged pores, and bacteria. Other common words we hear related to skin changes include: sebum, comedones, comedogenic, cysts, sebaceous glands, T-zone, inflammation, hair follicles, and the list goes on. Why is it important or helpful to know about all this scientific stuff? To a large extent, it isn't. People who are struggling with non-stop acne don't need to fixate on the nitty-gritty microscopic view of their pimples any more than someone with digestive upset needs to think about their mucosal lining and rugae. If you don't know what all these words mean, they're not important. The point is, knowing the terminology and the physical aspects of the bumps doesn't open doors to healing and resolving acne symptoms.

Medical experts, estheticians, nutritionists, and even T.V. commercials will tell you the opposite. They will imply that the more you know about your skin physically, the closer you are to stopping your acne for good. But they haven't found a cure using all their knowledge! With all the modern science and technology available today, if the experts had found a real solution to acne, we would have heard about it by now. Sometimes, pharmaceuticals and expensive skin care products can temporarily clear or alleviate symptoms while you're using (and paying for) them consistently. However, from my own experience and talking to patients about theirs, relying on any substance, whether chemical or natural, can become unsettling. We can get sick of being dependent on a crutch, annoyed at the time and cost involved in our regimens, and superstitious that if we quit the products, we're sure to be at the mercy of acne forever.

I'd like to avoid extremes and mention that acne treatments and products can be somewhat helpful toward bringing about clearer skin and alleviating self consciousness about breakouts. The skin care lines, cosmetics, and treatments we try can serve as a bridge toward getting us from point A—of uncontrollable acne—to point B, where acne is improved and not a huge focus in our lives. The problem becomes though, most people are not satisfied with using products as just a practical tool, and rather they are on the hunt for a permanent cure that doesn't exist out there in our world.

Because products seldom solve the problem, the main message that experts have for their patients or clients often boils down to the following: It's somehow your fault for failing to keep the bad bacteria away and not maintaining perfectly balanced hormones. If only you had a gluten- and dairy-free diet and stayed away from all processed and inflammatory foods. By the way, you're allergic to everything in your diet. If only you meditated regularly. If only you quit coffee and sugar for good. It's too bad you're not good at reducing your stress level down to 0. And unfortunately, your filtered water is not pure enough. Most likely your home environment is too toxic for your skin to be healthy. Finally, fruit is bad for your skin. I'm not suggesting that any of this is true, but my patients have come in to their first appointments upset that their health care providers had been giving them all of these messages. No joke.

Do you buy all of that?

I tried to follow recommendations like these when my acne was severe, and nothing clicked. Worse yet, the changes weren't sustainable for the long-term. Even if your food sensitivity test shows that you're allergic to everything under the sun, how long can you tolerate abstaining from all those foods in your diet? If you're constantly vigilant of toxins in your environment, what's to prevent you from going overboard and becoming hypersensitive and even anxious around all stimuli and molecules in the air? I personally couldn't maintain such a flawless and clean lifestyle and during my short bouts trying these methods, my skin didn't clear up or seem happier. In moderation, healthier habits did help me feel good overall. But my skin's response was not remarkable.

I've had patients who, prior to seeing me, overhauled their whole lives "correctly" as recommended by various health providers. Not only were these individuals still getting acne, but the lifestyle changes were also creating more stress than patients had felt when they were only dealing with breakouts. And with more lifestyle stress comes more skin stress. In certain cases, patients reported that their acne had only gotten worse with drastic changes to their life, even with those changes being supposedly healthier.

Much of the time the main triggers behind chronic acne are not physical ones like hormones, bacteria, sebum, or clogged pores. Yes, these are all part of the string of events leading up to a pimple or a breakout. But first, something has to start this chain reaction. In other words, the physical features are the effects, not the root causes of acne.

By treating acne like it's only a physical phenomenon, we're ignoring a simple but important fact—the body and mind exist together. Acne is shaped by our thoughts, our emotions, and also by social influences all around us. The high expectations and pressures that we face, ideals we're trying to live up to, and the drive to be perfect in this world all affect our skin. When we open up the door and head out into the world, the first thing people see and interact with is our face. Our skin is the boundary between us and the world. It's not just physical in nature, it's environmental and social as well.

We need a new playbook for acne, one that doesn't revolve around restrictive and stressful lifestyle changes. We also need a more creative approach that doesn't turn "solving the acne problem" into a way of life or a full-time job. People may try and convince you that this rigid mindset is the only way to get rid of our breakouts, but I haven't seen it work well yet. Do you really want to focus on acne all the time?

The truth is, acne is just another four-letter word. And when you boil it down, this vulgar little word is also just a *bully*.

What do I mean by this?....

Acne has a mean and nasty little personality, and it's trying to steal your energy and attention for itself by pushing you around.

Let me start by sharing a metaphor. Imagine that you are walking down the street and someone shoves you down to the ground. They start calling you names and disrespecting you. You get up and try to walk away, but this person follows you and keeps criticizing everything about you. They are not giving up. What would you do next? Would you invite them into a fancy restaurant and try to make them happy by ordering a five-course meal? Would you start paying them compliments and getting on their good side in the hopes that they leave you alone? Would you invite them to your home and rearrange everything there to accommodate your new guest? If you do all of that, it seems like this menacing person will stick around for good.

Acne is like that unwanted guest, and when we start flattering acne by changing our lives around for it, it actually gets comfortable and plans to stick around. This four-letter word is a relentless bully that is trying to run your life and tell you what to do. It curses you out on a daily basis and proclaims that you're weak against it, unable to do anything to make it go away. It gets in the way of things that you want, such as social interaction, putting yourself out there using your talents, and standing out as the unique person you are. It is trying to convince you that pimples are the most important thing in your life and that you should spend all your time getting to know them and solve them. It tells you that you are wrong and that you need to fix who you are. Wrong in what way? Just wrong. This little obscene word is being mean to you.

The mainstream health and skin care culture tells us to keep feeding the beast of acne by spending all our time and resources on appeasing it. Why are they giving us the runaround? Because they don't have the answers. The less people know about something, the more answers they provide about it. Have you noticed that? During my personal and professional experience treating acne, I haven't found one single answer either. I don't believe one exists for this symptom. But I have tried a different approach to handling this bully that gives skin a real chance to be healthy and clear. I've seen it work for myself and for patients who are open to doing one thing:

Standing up for themselves.

It's time to take back our lives. When we work around the clock for acne, we're playing into its hands by becoming invisible. It wants to overshadow you so that you fixate on it constantly. Eventually, all you see are the breakouts when you look in the mirror. You catalog where they are, how long they've been there, what products you've tried on them, and even how the pimples feel on a day to day basis. You might care less how you're doing than how your bumps are doing. Over time, it becomes more and more difficult to see yourself clearly for who you are. You wake up to acne, you go to bed with acne. Is this what you want?

Unfortunately, the acne solutions out there today are encouraging us to live in this manner. They add fuel to the fire of an already stressful lifestyle and mindset that stem from having acne. The skin care regimens, diets, and expert recommendations put acne at the center of your life and have you revolve around it. You spin around, and around, and around. And you arrive at the same spot. It's a tiring process that never acknowledges just how much acne is pushing you around. The acne solutions out there just shove you around even more.

Are you ready to leave the stressful safety of this hamster wheel and face the four-letter bully itself? The goal of this book is to help you do just that. No more running, no more hiding, not just from pimples, but from any influence in life that is feeding acne. By glaring right back at acne and making it clear that you're not going to put up with it, you unleash your innate potential for health and healing. The natural intelligence that your body already has for health is more powerful than any product, supplement, diet, and even pharmaceutical out there. And unlike acne treatments that are marketed as quick fixes, your body's own potential to promote clear skin costs no money and creates long-lasting change.

I can't guarantee that your acne will disappear within a set number of weeks or months once you start standing up to it. But you will be planting seeds of change that can take hold anytime. In my practice, I suggest natural therapies to patients in a limited way, emphasizing that the products are not the most important part of their treatment. Rather than focusing on what's being "taken," I spend most of my time with patients discussing the theme of this book: Acne is just another four-letter word, and it's time to stand up to it. To date, I've never had a patient say to me, "Thanks Dr. Patel—the natural supplement and skin moisturizer you recommended to me totally cured my acne." Patients who have seen their acne disappear use treatments simply as a tool for better skin health, but they don't seem reliant on them in any way.

Instead, patients will describe to me how acne just doesn't matter to them like it used to. They actively work on taking power away from the symptoms and giving it back to themselves. Increasingly with time, they assert a life away from this four-letter word until it can't bully them any longer. Have I or my patients known when this change will take place? No, but the regular practice of seeing acne as a mean and unwanted guest and standing up to it becomes the best medicine, and this new perspective makes real change possible.

Before we get started, I want to point out that this is not your typical book about acne. It doesn't cover ten regimented steps you can follow for better skin. I won't be outlining a 30-day plan for clearing up acne for good. The book won't encourage you to cut gluten, dairy, and sugar out of your diet for eternity. I also won't be describing certain lifestyle choices as "good" for your skin while other ones are "bad." The main point of this book is to see acne for what it is—a vulgar bully—and to stand up for yourself and separate your identity from it.

Society and mainstream healthcare suggest that we turn acne into a *very big deal* by actively fearing it and structuring our days around it. Their approach invites acne to grow into a bigger bully every day as we focus on its importance in our lives. The truth: All the fuss around acne is overblown and often inaccurate, and it just makes the situation worse. This book encourages you to make acne's role smaller in your life and to put the ball back in your court toward reclaiming your skin. You don't have to ditch your skin care products and treatments in order to benefit from this book. You can try whichever additional tools you want, and you may even find that they work better for you alongside the book, but the main power to stand up to acne and heal your skin will come from within you. Because of this, any benefits you experience will likely be long-lasting and not reliant on creams, capsules, or special diets for maintenance.

One important note: As you start standing up to acne, try and be patient and celebrate each progress no matter how small it is. The challenge behind acne is that people want to shift from having regular breakouts to wearing perfect skin overnight. I know the tendency, it's the same thing I wished for and that I hear patients in my office express. Despite the mind's push for flawless skin, we're going to take this process one step at a time and enjoy little successes whenever breakouts look or feel better.

If you don't give yourself credit for these little steps forward, it can become tempting to give up when your skin goes through backsliding or other challenges. Two steps forward, one step back is a common experience when you're trying to improve skin health. When you do celebrate progress forward, no matter how small, you build yourself a solid foundation to keep moving toward clear skin no matter which obstacles come along.

Next, let's take a closer look at what we mean by "bully" when we're describing acne. Acne isn't your garden variety bully that picks on people at the playground. That type of bully is overt in its behavior, and he or she often gets sent to the principal's office or is assigned detention as a result of how they treat others. The four-letter word we're dealing with is a different kind of menace, one that acts underneath the surface to try and undermine who we are. Let's call out the tricks that this bully tries to use on us.

CHAPTER 2

Hey, What Did You Just Say to Me?

———————•———————

In my naturopathic practice, I've noticed an interesting trend when seeing individuals who are dealing with acne. This trend unravels slowly as patients talk to me about their symptoms for the duration of an appointment. When they first sit down, everyone starts out by telling me the story of how acne entered their lives. It's amazing how much we can remember when it comes to acne's influence. Each patient will describe to me in detail the specific qualities of the bumps they're experiencing. They'll also recount numerous treatments they've tried out as well as a timeline about the ups and downs they've experienced with their skin.

During the early part of each patient's story, I'll hear bits and pieces of how this person was feeling when acne first showed up. I'll hear about the frustration that surfaced along with the acne, as well as anxiety, anger, and fear that it would never go away. The next part of the story is very different. As I talk to patients more in-depth about the treatments they've tried out and the roller coaster timeline of acne's intensity in their lives, their tone usually shifts. All of a sudden, I'm hearing from my patient one, and only one cause of acne.

Over time, I've learned to loosen the doctor's hat I'm wearing so that I can hear what patients are really implying is the root of their acne. Clinically, I'll hear about my patients' dietary habits, their newest face wash and moisturizer, digestive health, and how much they're sleeping at night. You know, the typical questions that you get asked at the doctor's office. When I first started out in practice, I was looking for trends in how patients were answering these questions. I made check marks all over the place next to their answers and looked for a physical cause to their skin issues.

The trend I was looking for just wasn't showing up. Patients with typically "healthy" diets had as much trouble with acne as those with typically "unhealthy" diets. I had patients who exercised and those who didn't. Laid back type B individuals and higher strung type A ones. Those who went to bed early and those who were night owls. Some were gluten- and dairy-free, and others seemed to live on bread and cheese. I had patients who swore by supplements and other ones who didn't care for them. What about their skin care habits? Patients used just about anything, ranging from over-the-counter products to high end skin care lines.

My investigative zeal was deflating the more I relied strictly on my doctor's hat. I wasn't gathering enough useful clues to help patients, and that frustrated me. It must have been one such moment of frustration during a patient visit when I stopped in my tracks. I still listened to the actual words my patient was sharing with me, but I also started listening behind those words. I had experienced years of acne myself, so it wasn't too difficult for me to switch the frequency and tune in to a different voice I was hearing tell the story. What was the one underlying cause of acne according to this patient, and to others who I talked to after that day?

They felt they were doing something wrong.

In patients' minds, they were somehow to blame for this whole ordeal. At some point, they stopped looking for a cure for acne and instead embarked on a quest to find and categorize everything they were doing wrong with their skin—and their lives. On the surface it looked like it was all about acne, but underneath, the feeling of wrongness was pervasive and not focused on the skin alone. The more I listened to patients tell their stories and remembered my own, I had to ask whether the chicken came first or the egg. Did people feel wrong because they felt personally responsible for the bumps on their skin? Or did they feel wrong before acne ever came along?

In an overt way, acne physically bullies you using bumps, redness, and irritation. It is persistent and it affects your appearance on a regular basis. It glares right at you in the mirror. But acne isn't just a look. If you listen carefully, acne has a voice that keeps saying one thing over and over again: You're wrong . . . you're wrong . . . you're wrong. *You're wrong for being who you are.* Even though unsightly bumps seem like the worst part of acne, they're not the main tactic that acne uses to bully someone. The message that this four-letter word keeps yelling at us is more detrimental than the breakouts themselves.

Step one in facing acne: Recognize the words and messages it's using against you.

How do we uncover the obscenities that this four-letter word keeps sending our way? The truth is, we already know about the insulting things acne says to us. We live with the words and self-defeating messages on a daily basis. The main challenge lies in people's desire to ignore what they're hearing. It's not comfortable to admit to yourself that you feel wrong for being who you are. So we spend a lot of time trying to act like we don't feel this way and that all we care about is fixing our appearance and being acne-free.

Everyone deals with the challenge of feeling wrong as they are at times. Even though most doctors won't acknowledge how this feeling can affect health—in fact, some docs may even jump on the bandwagon in making their patients feel they are doing something wrong—this is a real factor that can affect the functioning of the body. For those dealing with acne, this struggle rises to the surface and appears on the skin itself. For others, it can disrupt health in a variety of ways such as upsetting digestion, causing weight gain, prompting anxiety, leading to insomnia, or triggering allergies, for example.

Because acne sits on the skin for everyone *out there* to notice, those of us dealing with it may try even harder to suppress any feelings we have about not looking or acting "right." We don't want anyone to see this insecurity, especially since they already can see the acne itself. Remember how I mentioned earlier that acne isn't a typical bully in the way it behaves? It is sneakier than the typical bully who dishes out mistreatment and humiliation in public. Acne will tell you that you're wrong for being who you are, but it accomplishes this by *convincing you that these words are your own.* Eventually, you start echoing this voice because you mistakenly think it's the only one you have.

Step two in facing acne: Separate your voice from the four-letter bully's voice.

Many of us dealing with acne become trapped with the misconception that we feel inherently wrong, and that we're just born this way. This is acne's voice, not yours. Where did acne get this voice from? We'll soon talk about this more in-depth, but for now what's important to see is that acne is a physical manifestation of external influences. Its voice isn't the same as your own, and what acne is doing is parroting the voices you have heard around you while growing up and going through life.

When you start paying more attention to these messages and hear them clearly, you may realize that they're not very different from the thoughts you have when staring at acne in the mirror:

You don't look right.
Don't show yourself to the world.
Stay inside and hide your face.
Who's going to believe anything you say or do?
Don't bother taking yourself seriously, it's not worth it.
Just give up, these bumps will be here forever.
Other people look good, and they deserve to be seen instead of you.
You need help, but nothing will be able to fix this problem no matter where you search.

Look at that pimple, look at that pimple, look at that pimple. Look at you doing it all wrong.

Why can't you just look and act normal, like other people?

This isn't good enough. Do better and do more. Stop trying to do it your way.

Does any of this sound familiar? If so, you're not alone. The more patients I've seen for acne in my office, the more I've heard these self-defeating words echoed in patient stories and recognized them clearly from my own experience. These messages can be so confusing for people, because deep down they do care about themselves, their health, and their appearance. But acne will always scream its obscenities back at us and try to make us forget what matters to us most.

Once I ask my patients to share their experiences, I find that many of them are very aware of how they're feeling about acne and what they're going through. It just hasn't been easy for them to let these insights come to the surface in everyday life. It's common that when patients start to touch on their own feelings and thoughts regarding acne, they'll very often hear advice from a health provider, friend, or family member along the lines of, "Just cut out gluten and everything will get resolved." Or, "Sugar is bad, eliminate that from your diet. Your face wash and moisturizer need to be more organic and non-toxic. Wash your pillow case and don't touch your face. Your pores are too big, you may want to exfoliate. Try an electronic cleansing brush."

The list of tips and advice goes on and on. It's always about *doing more* instead of paying attention to your own voice underneath that's shouting out to be heard. After exposure to these prescriptive tidbits, patients easily lose touch with their own voices and get back to nit picking their skin and lifestyle habits. They also get back to staring in the mirror 24/7, fixating on each pimple's life course and everything that is wrong.

Acne's voice is not original or unique. Nothing it's saying to you is important, even though it's trying to adopt a tone of authority in your life and over your skin. When it tells you to stare at your pimples in detail, it's just taking your attention off of your life and how you're doing and instead putting it onto itself. Acne eventually becomes not only a bullying influence, but also a huge distraction from what matters to you in your life.

Step three in facing acne: Turn to it and ask, "Hey, what did you just say to me?"

This four-letter word thinks it can keep getting away with the yelling, obscenities, insults, and casually belittling remarks. It bides its time, relying on you to keep the dynamic going for fear of something bad happening if you don't. It's a patient beast, but at the end of the day the messages it's sending your way are as puny as the pimples behind which it speaks. It may be heard to believe that I'm describing acne's bullying voice as weak and unimportant. After all, it's creating all this mayhem and distress for you on a daily basis, right? It's relentless and seems to show no mercy. Yet, I maintain that it's powerless when standing face to face with you. I'll tell you why:

It's wrong.

Deep down, the message this voice keeps repeating over and over doesn't sit right with you. Just like patients I've seen in my office, you may share in common the feeling that you're doing it all wrong, especially when you're listening to the voice of acne. However, just like my patients, you may feel confused about what exactly you're doing wrong. *That's because you're not wrong, and that voice is.* And that's a fact. Even though this is a fact, it's not an easy one to accept. I don't have to double check before telling you that there are no peer-reviewed research articles out there confirming that, scientifically speaking, acne is wrong in the message it's sending to you. That is not the type of research that pharmaceutical companies, insurance systems, mainstream medicine, or the skin care industry is interested in. It doesn't sell anything for them.

However, you can do this type of research and experiment with it in your own life with greater results. In your gut, you may already feel what I'm talking about when I say acne is wrong. If so, the next step is not running from the nasty insults you're hearing, but instead questioning acne on exactly what it's saying. Time to start calling out what this bully is implying about you in the mirror.

When you start to face the insults acne is throwing at you, you'll recognize them as familiar foes. Acne is simply the hired muscle and sidekick for external influences already present in your life, which have been trying to tell you who you are. The bumps themselves are a physical representation of feeling watched, scrutinized, and criticized in an unfair way. You know who you are, but the messages acne keeps sending are meant to convince you that you're wrong. Instead, they claim that other people see you better than you see yourself. They know who you really are, and you don't.

You may have adopted similar sounding messages for yourself over time, especially while dealing with acne. *But these thoughts aren't born from you.* The more you practice calling out acne and all its swear words, the more natural it will be for you to separate your own voice from this bullying one. As this occurs, the skin can start reclaiming its integrity and resilience. Over time, you can feel more comfortable living in and enjoying your skin—not just on a physical level, but throughout your life.

Next, we'll look more in-depth at the specific messages acne tends to use, so that it becomes easier to call them out. Acne has many ways that it likes to push our buttons and keep us involved in its drama. It knows that you want to be left alone, so it fires obscenities from different directions in an attempt to never leave you alone. The diverse insults acne uses are related to each other and have the same goal in harassing you, but it's still important to recognize all of them for what they are. The bully rewords its messages to make you think it's delivering a new put-down every time, so that you'll listen. As you learn to catch it red-handed no matter which message it's using, the less creative acne can be in poking at you.

CHAPTER 3

Now, Just Be a Good Little Girl (or Boy)

———————— • ————————

For many, acne first surfaces during the teenage years. This is a time when kids start becoming young adults and asserting their own voices and authority out in the world. They take footsteps out into the unknown that may look shaky, but are also solid steps of independence and expression as a unique individual. Is it any wonder that the four-letter bully we're dealing with, the one that tries to be a false authority over us, often starts to appear right when we're wanting to courageously head out into our blossoming lives? This bully tries to stand in the way of a natural growth that someone is trying to go through in life.

It's easy to think of acne as just a "teenage thing," but it doesn't shake off so easily for everyone after the teenage years. Increasingly, more adults are also facing acne, sometimes for the first time in their lives. Understandably, they wonder why these symptoms are surfacing for them. The bumps immediately make anyone wearing them, of any age, look younger, more inexperienced, and exposed in a disconcerting way.

We feel like little girls or boys again, like someone who is years away from growing up. We don't have the protective barrier up that we need between us and the outside world and our skin feels like it's betraying us. We take a time machine right back to middle school or high school, when everyone thinks they can tell you what to do. What does acne ultimately make someone feel?

Acne makes you feel like you're in trouble.

Even though the phrase "in trouble" is connected with being a kid, everyone feels in trouble at times. It is not a feeling that can be completely outgrown once you stop being grounded by your parents or sent to your room without dessert. We imagine that there is a "right" way to do things, and we don't want to be caught doing things the "wrong" way. We're not quite sure who is the ultimate judge that determines right from wrong, but we know that these expectations are out there and we're naturally affected by them because we're human. We become tuned in to what friends, family, and other people seem to be saying about us, and whether they approve of what we're doing as "right." Life can fill up with demands of "I should" at every turn, and we may put tons of effort into not getting in trouble (or more trouble than we feel we're already in).

One of the most common bullying tactics acne uses is yelling out that you're in terrible, one-of-a-kind, humiliating, irreparable trouble—all the time. It declares that there's probably nothing you can do about it, but maybe if you try harder, you'll have a small chance of reversing your bad fortune of being so bad. It constantly says:

Now, just be a good little girl or boy.

Of course, acne is imitating a voice that we're already used to hearing in society, and that is why this bullying tactic is so effective. Whether it's coming from our upbringing, a strict teacher's classroom, an uptight medical office, a friend, a workplace, or any other environment, most of us are familiar with the Be Good message. Taken to the extreme, this message is not at all what it seems. While the sentiment may sound caring on the surface, as if it's meant to help you or teach you something, it's anything but caring underneath. Its main point is that you should strive extremely hard to be someone who you're not. Be Good means: You're bad. Fall in line, or you're in trouble. This is the demand that acne places on us, both through physical harassment on our skin and through parroting a voice common in society that tells us to blindly obey.

22

There doesn't even have to be someone in your environment always reminding you to be good. Soon enough, we start treating ourselves like a little kid who is in trouble all the time. An imaginary police figure in the mind starts watching and tracking what we do and say on a daily basis. Acne happens to be a symptom that makes someone feel like they're under a microscope in front of people, and it's no coincidence that the mind is placing that same person under a microscope for who they are.

Mainstream skin care experts often point out the common feelings someone develops after acne surfaces. These include insecurity, doubt, and feeling unfairly watched and judged. But what if most people are already feeling excessively watched and scrutinized before acne ever starts? Like we talked about earlier and will explore more throughout the book, it's a question of the chicken or the egg. It's easy to attribute what someone's going through *after* acne occurs as simply a result or effect of the physical symptoms. This isn't the full story though. Acne, a harsh and bullying symptom, is an expert imitator of challenging and often harsh circumstances that *already* exist. One of these is the constant feeling of being watched and in trouble.

When we're trying treatment after treatment, product after product, and bending over backwards to soothe acne's chronic and unpredictable temper tantrums—are we always doing it with the real belief our skin will get healthier? For many people, the process of treating breakouts includes a huge element of panic and fear. When we wake up and see acne in the mirror, it's almost like it's staring at us more than we're looking at it. You want to yell, "Stop watching me!" And if you have other areas in your life where you feel watched and judged, this desire to stop being scrutinized and criticized is more than just skin-deep.

We throw products and treatments at acne almost like ammunition, wanting to hurt it on the one hand and if that's not possible, calm it down toward relative peace with your skin. It's not the actual topical cream or medicine you're using that's the problem, however. When acne thinks it has authority over us and we're constantly checking in to see whether it is appeased by a new product, it will use whatever power and attention we're giving it to bully us. It continues to stick around to watch, police, and judge. It knows that you're trying to be good and bend to its needs, and it gives you a default label of "bad" that you have to battle against.

The stress of being watched by acne only adds to the stress we're already feeling while trying to be good and while bobbing and weaving the label of "bad." Of course, stress in the body only contributes more to acne breakouts and a cycle quickly develops. Acne doesn't stop there in its effect on the body. In our society, feelings of happiness and joy are typically seen as positive feelings while other honest emotions like frustration, anger, anxiety, and insecurity come to be seen as negative or bad. This makes many people want to project more happiness in favor of other emotions, whether they're really feeling that way or not. It's natural for the body to process other emotions too, and people dealing with acne experience a variety of feelings both before and after breakouts surface.

Imagine if you have to stuff down all your frustration and anxiety while dealing with acne. Yet, that's exactly what this bully demands from you while it's urging you to be a good girl or boy. If you're not feeling happy, that's considered bad according to acne and any other social influences that its borrowing insulting messages from.

We may ignore our natural responses in hopes that they go away, but they remain in our bodies, trapped under the surface and contributing to our skin issues. The suppression of less than happy emotions makes acne symptoms worse than if the body were allowed to process these feelings naturally. This connection in skin health is so important that I'll devote a whole chapter to it later. For now, just keep in mind that acne insults us not only with its bullying tactics, but also by telling us that *we're not allowed to have a response* to this bad treatment.

The voice that watches and judges you, from acne and its related influences, is not your own. It may feel at times like this voice is born from you and describes accurately how you view yourself, but it's actually separate from you. Watching and policing is one of the main tricks acne uses to push you around. Acne tries to convince you that it's important to watch every move you make until you catch yourself red-handed doing something wrong. Meanwhile, it becomes more and more difficult to move at all.

Where can you go when you fear that each move you make, each step you take, and every word you voice will be wrong and bad? Acne's message implies that it's directing you on a better and safer path, one that protects you from getting in deep water and regretting your actions. It claims it will teach you how to make a better impression on others in the long-run. It will teach you to do the right thing, to be a good little girl or boy. What it's really doing, however, is stopping you.

Who does acne think it is? What right does it have to watch and judge us?

Step four in facing acne: Question its authority to police your skin and your life.

Before you lift another finger trying to shift your life, health, and skin care routine around for acne, ask yourself what is driving your actions. Naturally, you'll want to experiment to see what helps your skin feel better. However, if you feel compelled to make changes out of fear, panic, or not wanting acne to be angry at you, the efforts you're making will be stopped in their tracks. The focus will shift toward a frantic desire to avoid "getting in trouble" with your skin's breakouts. You end up taking care of acne's strict commands rather than attending to yourself and your skin.

For many of my patients who first describe their acne to me, there is a recurrent theme of running in circles trying so many different things to make acne happy so it stops picking on them. Patients don't feel involved in the process personally, and it's almost as if their decisions are a form of damage control. They get in the habit of trying to dodge whatever bad thing may happen, both on their skin and in life overall.

You don't have to be good all the time to move toward clearer skin. In fact, if you really want to tell acne off, it's helpful to break from the "be good" cycle that it's demanding from you. You don't have to find the perfect face wash or moisturizer to appease acne. It's also not necessary to cut every so-called bad food out of your diet and eat 100% clean (whatever that means). You can skip juicing all your fruits and vegetables, applying harsh medicated products, and taking ten different supplements and herbs—if you don't want to. What you're left with is following your instinct toward any changes that you really *want to* make. Not because you have to according to acne and its fear-mongering, but because you feel like doing it for yourself.

At the same time, it's helpful to question other influences in your life that may be making you feel like acne is trying to make you feel: bad, and in trouble all the time. Any social dynamics around you that are watchful and unfairly judgmental may be long-standing, and for that reason they can be challenging to look at for what they are. Like I mentioned earlier, it's common to hear messages from people you know that sound caring on the surface, yet that possess an undertone of "You're bad and in trouble. Now fall in line like you're supposed to, or else..." If anyone is trying to make you feel this way using a falsely authoritative voice, then maybe that person is being bad—not you.

So, regardless of what acne tries to tell you to your face, *you don't have acne because you're bad and deserving of punishment.* You're also not breaking out because you're doing all the wrong things with your lifestyle and day-to-day routines. We naturally want to feel confident in any health measures we're taking in our lives, and that can be a challenge when acne keeps shoving its agenda into our earnest efforts to get clearer skin. Many of my patients try out a new product or skin technique for a week or two before ditching it. On the opposite end of the spectrum, they also tend to endure extreme dietary changes or skin care routines for long periods of time, even when the techniques aren't working to clear up acne. There is a feeling of "I *should* stick with this" that enters their minds, and patients will feel very concerned if they break from a regimen, even if it's ineffective and incompatible with daily life. I'm no stranger to this pattern from my own history with acne.

Why is there such a strong feeling of worry surrounding health and skin care habits when you have acne? Worry typically stems from a feeling that there is a right way and a wrong way to do something, and when you have acne you don't want to accidentally stumble on the wrong path and make it worse. On the surface, it makes sense that you'd want to strike gold on finding the right acne treatment to end breakouts for good. The truth is however, even though we want to believe all our decisions regarding acne are rational, this isn't always the case. Acne knows about the worry, fear, and indecisiveness that runs through our minds when we break out. And it loves to play on these thoughts—big time. It toys with us, like a cat would with a mouse. It makes us doubt everything we do.

Yes, there is a unique path you can take for effectively healing your acne, one that fits who you are. But whatever you do, don't ask acne what that path should involve, because it only wants to steer you in the wrong direction.

CHAPTER 4

Cross Your Fingers, and Maybe Someday...

———————•———————

S ome people like to find head's up pennies on the ground because they think it's a sign of good luck. Others won't step on cracks in the sidewalk because they don't want any bad luck that they believe is associated with that. It's hard to pinpoint where superstitions come from in the first place, but in small doses, they're not so bad. They can even make daily life interesting and fun at times. When taken to extremes or allowed to rule daily life, however, superstitions typically stop being fun. The superstitious voice that acne uses against us is not the lighthearted kind, and it often becomes a debilitating force in the life of someone who is already dealing with chronic breakouts. It tries to make us believe that every little thing we do, think, or say may somehow lead to pimples.

For many, acne also carries with it a sense of bad luck that they may not even be aware of. It may feel as if you're cursed or that life is against you, and that you have little or no control over this trend. When each breakout occurs, it just becomes another piece of evidence that nothing is going your way, and this way of thinking can become a cycle. You come to expect pimples as a matter of course, regardless of what efforts you're putting forth to get rid of them. The bad luck can start to become a self-fulfilling prophecy. When it comes to the stories surrounding our skin or anything else that matters to us, we might eventually stop hoping for much good to come out of it.

But the story is still being written, and it's easy to forget this while acne is plaguing us with superstitions. This four-letter word already started its mistreatment by telling us that we're inherently bad and that we need to try extra hard to be good. On top of that, it adds a maddening level of hocus pocus to our existing skin woes. Acne tries to make you believe that these superstitions will eventually help your skin get better, but instead they only draw attention away from what you're really going through underneath the breakouts. It's yet another trick acne uses to distract you from your life and who you are. It can turn acne into a pseudo-religion in your life, one in which pimples decide your fate for you, rather than you having any say in how you want to live.

In the moment, the superstitions related to acne may sound very sane and rational. When you see the first signs of a pimple surfacing, you might feel some panic and helplessness. Then your mind quickly shifts to problem-solving mode. Naturally, you want to soothe or alleviate your skin's distress in some way, and this is a normal reaction. But acne has tied its hocus pocus into your natural instincts, so it can be difficult to tease apart the superstitions from any healthy intentions you're having toward your skin. After acne has been whispering these superstitions into your ear long enough, you may even find yourself seeking out irrational fixes for your skin over any practical approaches.

Everything you do can get lumped into the pseudo-religion of acne. What was once just a new skin care product that you were trying, or a treatment recommended by a trusted health care provider, can become a crutch you're dependent on. You may find it increasingly difficult to establish a healthy distance between you and the different tools you're using to treat your acne. Instead of just being a topical cream, zit-zapper, or cosmetic, a product can become a talisman that you feel you can't live without. When the products aren't effective, you may feel like it's another sign of bad luck and that the universe is against you.

Over time, the superstitions can invade your diet, leisure time, social events, education, career, relationships, or anything else that matters to you. Acne's bullying doesn't just stop at the skin. It wants to radiate its effects outward into your whole life. Acne urges you to stop thinking for yourself, and instead it wants you to close your eyes and believe the following message:

Cross your fingers, and maybe I'll leave you alone someday.

Every day, people dealing with acne wonder if "someday" has arrived yet, and they are often disappointed to learn that it hasn't. Meanwhile, they've been crossing their fingers just as acne's been telling them to do. Instead of allowing themselves to let loose and enjoy the day, people may find themselves following a set of subliminal instructions constantly sent to them by acne. The little tidbits of "advice" never seem to stop, and though they may seem relatively harmless on the surface, they are ultimately trying to tell you how to live. This superstitious voice can also be incredibly maddening! It may sound like:

I have to apply exactly three drops of facial cream, or else I'll break out. Oh no, I think I used four, now I'm going to get a pimple. I should use the cream three times per day. Oh no, I think I only did it twice yesterday, now I'm going to get even more pimples!

These cookies say they're gluten-free, which is good for my skin, but what if there's still gluten in there somewhere?

Is all my makeup off? Maybe I should wash my face a few more times.

My friend told me my skin looks good today. I'm scared now that a breakout is coming soon, and it will mess everything all up.

I noticed that when I ate popcorn the other day, I got acne soon after. I'm not eating popcorn anymore.

Sweating on that treadmill might aggravate my skin. I'll skip exercise just in case.

I need to get exactly eight hours of sleep, on the dot. If I don't, my acne will get worse.

Did I break out less when I wore that purple shirt, and more when I wore that red one?

I'm going to cross my fingers that I don't have zits tomorrow when I get my picture taken.

The superstitious voice of acne can make someone's world feel smaller and smaller, until they feel trapped and unable to confidently venture out into new and unexplored territory. This bullying tactic is meant to make you perpetually scared of the unknown, and even of the known. All of a sudden, you can't go to a party or other social gathering without worrying how the food there is going to mess with your skin. You can become hyperaware of all your routines and actions, not wanting to step on an invisible bomb that will set off more acne. For many, anxiety will rise from the heightened fear and superstition, which only seems to make acne worse.

Again, we have to revisit the question of the chicken or the egg: Do we feel unlucky only because acne won't go away? Maybe the feeling of being unlucky, cursed, or trapped by superstitions was present to some extent before acne surfaced, and now this four-letter word is simply taking advantage of those circumstances.

When working with patients who are dealing with acne, I will often hear about long-standing influences in their lives that have been trying to stifle their confidence and freedom to make independent decisions. These voices will suggest that the patient can't trust his or her own instinct and direction in life. When someone feels constantly pressured to give up pursuing what they want, or that person is made to feel silly or foolish for wanting anything in the first place, it's easy to feel at the mercy of the universe. All of a sudden, your actions don't seem to matter, and instead the world gets to decide what should happen to you. You're either lucky, or not. And acne keeps hammering the message that you better cross your fingers, because it's not looking good for you. Acne acts like it's deciding your reality for you, and you have no choice in the matter.

The superstitions can start to invade any attempts you make toward going for what you want, even outside of your desire to get rid of acne. These thoughts can sound like:

I'll apply for that scholarship, but I don't stand a chance of getting it because of who I am.

Even if I apply for jobs, I know the world is against me and no employer will get back to me.

I wish I could get excited about what I really want in life, but I'm too unlucky to ever reach that point.

People are right about me that I don't have what it takes. Why do I bother?

It's not only people with acne who have these thoughts and feelings. But for those who are plagued by this four-letter word, the signs of apparent bad luck are visible on the skin in the form of zits, which serve as a constant reminder that the curse is hanging around. Even when my patients notice some success in clearing up their skin, they often feel superstitious that these steps forward will eventually be yanked backward by acne. Acne becomes the only reality, along with any other influences in life that act belittling, cursing, and all-knowing. These bullies ask you to worship them and dance in fearful circles for them, instead of paying attention to what matters to you in your life.

The things that you want in life and that are important to you don't go away though, no matter how much acne tries to shrink your world and take you away from them. Instead of letting pimples have their way, we can try dwarfing their size and influence by prioritizing real life ahead of them.

Step five in facing acne: Live your life anyway.

The worst insult to acne is to live your life, right in the face of its hocus pocus, arbitrary rules, and backward magic. Little by little, you can practice uncrossing your fingers when taking care of your skin. This small practice will naturally extend to other things in your life as well, such as career, education, family life, hobbies, social interaction, or anything else you're putting energy toward.

At first, your mind may ridicule you by stating: Living life without these superstitions is too risky, and sounds easier said than done. That's okay, try to say it and do it. On days when it feels challenging to dodge the superstitions, you can still remind yourself that the arbitrary rules aren't all powerful and important like they act. These superstitions are not based in reality and instead are rooted in false ideas. Acne's weaker than you think, and it'll show its weakness when you take steps toward directing, owning, and connecting with your life. As you gradually make it a habit to kick skin-related superstitions to the curb, acne will say, "Oh no—I'm losing influence here. He (or she) isn't jumping to my whims as much."

Acne wants to bully you into believing that your luck will nosedive if you try to get rid of this four-letter word. In a twisted way, it wants you to think it's your only stab at having luck enter your life. It wants you to cross your fingers and wait. Wait for perfect skin, wait for all the pimples to go away. Then, maybe you can start to live your life. As we wait, life goes on and we often miss real opportunities that come along or that we can pursue. Meanwhile, acne keeps insisting, "Hey, you don't have much sense, luck, or confidence when it comes to your life. But at least you can control your little routines and superstitions around breakouts."

We can easily get hooked on these acne-based routines and superstitions as if they're our life savers instead of being little curses that acne keeps branding us with. My patients are often surprised to discover that they're scared at the prospect of *not having* acne around in their lives. They'll often meet up with this fear when they make progress toward clearing up their skin. They're scared not to have control over what will happen once acne clears up. They'll stand out for having clearer skin, and that's venturing into the unknown. What will others think? What new opportunities will come along, and will they be ready for them after identifying with acne for so long? Being acne-free is unfamiliar to people who are dealing with breakouts, but living with acne's cursing voice is very familiar, controllable in its routine, and therefore, almost comforting.

I encourage patients, and you, to start messing with this familiarity and put a wrench in acne's plans. When acne's trying to invoke its spells, even little interruptions can make a difference. I'll ask patients to experiment a bit with their skin care routines instead of sticking with the regimens and amounts of product they're habitually used to. I'll even tell a patient to skip part of their routine for just a day, for example going one morning without a face wash they're hooked on. Just splash a little water on your face instead. Guess what? Nothing bad happens and life moves on. You'll start to see that your skin's mood and health don't hinge on a small routine or superstition that you've built around acne.

You can also eat a square of chocolate if you've been staying away from it, or maybe dabble with some gluten or dairy that has stayed forbidden in your life. Go ahead and stay up a little later to enjoy the nighttime if you don't want acne to strictly enforce your bedtime. Leave your hair down and let it touch your skin, even if acne's been telling you it's superstitiously bad to do so. It's okay to let loose and show acne you're not afraid to have fun. Nothing bad is going to happen, you tell it, from me doing and getting what I want.

Try adding a creative twist when applying your makeup, or experiment with a new look or hairstyle. Acne doesn't own your appearance, you do. Practice stepping out of your comfort zone and challenging yourself to defy acne's hang ups that it's trying to pass onto you. If you break out, don't worry. You're stepping out of your comfort zone, and it can be a bit scary at first to try something new. Over time, you'll develop more confidence surrounding whatever steps you're taking, and this boost in confidence is protective against acne.

Life's not going to punish or hurt you just because you enjoy, engage in, and appreciate your life. In fact, you will most likely see rewards sprouting from letting yourself do these things. Acne just uses its superstitious voice to try and make you believe it's the opposite. The more you warm up to the reality of the situation and see acne's agenda for what it is, the more you can move forward in your life, and in supporting the health of your skin.

With that mindset, you can also take small steps toward an activity, hobby, or skill that has felt off limits due to acne's harassment. Maybe there's a new direction you've wanted to take in your career, and it's been scary to pursue up to now. It could be you've been eyeing a sport or exercise that has fallen to the backburner. You may have creative interests that have felt out of reach. Perhaps you're not quite ready to act yet, but you want the freedom to think about what makes you feel excited and engages your energy. Over time, you can try taking new risks and letting your talents and ability shine, much like in the way you'd like your skin to radiate who you are over time.

Your skin's clarity might not change significantly in the moment, but with less fear and anxiety surrounding your actions going forward, the symptoms will have a less cluttered path toward getting better. Step by step, you can get more comfortable in your skin, your day, and your life. In the process, you get less comfortable with the familiar and superstitious voice of acne. Of course, insecurities and fears around your skin may come up from time to time, but they don't have to rule everything you do and feel.

When someone sends me an update to say their skin is looking and feeling better, there's always more to the story. I'll hear about ways in which people are venturing into new territory in other areas of life too. Someone I worked with became more invested in her dream to pursue performance dance. Another individual realized she was taking care of others so much, she had forgotten her own health. She then shifted more focus onto herself and was experiencing less stress and more energy toward her life. A freshman college student gained the confidence to meet new people in her classes and extracurricular activities. The benefit from disrupting acne's superstitions isn't only skin deep, it radiates outward into your life. And no matter what anyone says, you can't buy that in a skin care product or treatment—regardless of the superstitious sounding sales pitch someone is using to market it to you.

Your actions matter and make a real difference, not acne's hurtful and irrational words. Uncrossing your fingers helps you pave the way for your own luck, appreciate what you already have in life, and remember who you are apart from acne. It unlocks your innate courage and confidence, and it lets you venture into the unknown as the person you already are.

Feeling comfortable in your own skin renews its strength and is naturally protective against breakouts over the long-term. Acne will front like it can mess all that up for you with a bunch of petty superstitions, but you don't have to believe it. This bully doesn't stand a chance as long as you recognize the fear tactics it uses and call out its cowardice for what it is.

CHAPTER 5
Give in to the Nothing

I t's common for those of us with acne to feel like our skin is betraying us by allowing pimples to invade our lives. We may then want to attack our skin, and since the skin is a part of us, we end up attacking ourselves too. Even though you see acne reflected in the mirror, I assure you that *your skin isn't against you.* It's built to protect you, reflect who you are, and give you healthy distance from the world around you.

Your skin has three specific jobs that it's performing right now as we speak. It's serving as a natural boundary between you and the environment. It's helping you regulate your body temperature by adjusting its blood supply. Finally, it's sensing stimulus for you in the environment, including heat, cold, pressure, contact, and pain. Clearly, the skin is important as it's the largest organ in the body. One of its major roles is to sense, so the skin actually feels things for you— literally.

It's easy to notice sensations on the skin that cause reactions like "ouch" or "that feels good." In a given day, there are many different feelings the skin can experience on the surface. For those with acne, that daily experience includes the sensitivity, throbbing, irritation, and heat that comes with pimples. Put together with the effect acne has on our appearance, these sensations can become a real nuisance and distraction. We may even pay extra attention to how pimples feel in order to gauge when the next one's coming, and to try and predict when a breakout will ease up its bullying. A lot of our focus lies on the surface of how acne looks and feels.

The skin is a boundary, however, so by definition it's surrounded by both external and internal environments. Right now, your skin is doing its job of sensing surface stimuli (or close to the surface when it comes to pimples), but it's also sensing the inner environment of your body. It communicates with and responds to the hormones, neurotransmitters, and other physiological molecules that function every day to support life. These molecules are also chemical messengers that communicate and process how we're feeling.

While the surface of our skin keeps demanding constant attention due to the pain and rude appearance of acne, it's easy to forget the other side. What is the skin feeling inwardly? This question connects with another important question:

What is the person feeling?

The skin, and therefore you, experience acne both on the surface and well before it ever reaches there. The skin forms a network with the rest of the body, and its internal connections are just as important as its outward role in your life. Your skin can sense how you're feeling *in there*, which includes your emotions, stress, and fears. This is a normal and healthy function of the skin, and those emotions are normal and healthy reactions to living life. As usual, acne enjoys bullying you by attacking anything that is natural and healthy in your life, and so it goes after your very real responses to being human. It tries to suppress your emotions, and it gets you to do the dirty work for it.

What—now acne won't even let us be human? Acne's a very extreme bully, as you've probably noticed. Do you ever feel like acne makes you feel somewhat invisible? If so, you're not alone. This is a very common feeling for those with acne. All the attention we may get from the bumps on our face doesn't make us feel good, and ironically it can make us feel like no one really sees us. It's like we're disappearing behind the attention grubbing breakouts. On the opposite side of our skin to where acne lives, acne encourages us to deny our emotions and make us invisible to ourselves too. The silencing of important feelings undermines the skin's health, our expression as unique individuals, and our lives. All the while, acne applauds. It knows that suppressed emotions can trigger and aggravate the physical symptoms on your skin. With each breakout, acne tries to hit home the cruel message:

You don't exist.

How does the skin take a hit when we ignore our real feelings? Let's use a metaphor to take a look at what happens underneath your skin. Imagine trying to get in touch with people you know and not hearing anything back. You're using phone, e-mail, text, social media, and even snail mail to get someone, anyone, to respond. You wait patiently, and eventually you start feeling panic set in from the lack of response. You keep reaching out to others anyway and as time goes on, the phone messages you've left, e-mails you've written out, messages you've texted, and any other communications start backing up. The letters you've written are appearing in your own mailbox, marked "Return to Sender." Your e-mails are coming back too, with error messages attached to them.

You naturally start wondering where everyone has gone, and are frustrated that no one cares about your attempts at communicating. People know you and you have a history with them, so it doesn't make sense that they wouldn't acknowledge that connection by getting back to you. Some of the messages you sent were about challenging times you went through. Others allowed you to vent about situations that made you feel angry or anxious. You also had some good news to share, about exciting changes in your life or new opportunities that you'd been waiting for. Because no one is responding, it starts feeling like no one knows you anymore. You even start to question whether you feel as in touch with who you are.

Regardless, you continue to send out messages to people you know, with a little hope remaining that someone will talk to you eventually. Some of the wind has gone out of your sails, but it's worth it to you to keep trying. Still, nothing happens. This backed up communication becomes like gunk in your life. It's hard to process what you're going through with all of the rejected messages sitting around. Unfortunately, these messages aren't easy to delete or get rid of either. You try to ignore them as much as you can, but they're cluttering your space. They're slowly blocking you from connecting with your health, and your life, and it's discouraging you from expressing or doing anything moving forward. After a while of this cycle, you don't care as much anymore. You try and paste a smile on your face and pretend like nothing's wrong, but inwardly it's irking you that no one out there cares. Worse yet, whether you acknowledge it or not, it bothers you that you've stopped caring.

In real life, you don't have ultimate control over how other people communicate with you, but you do have the opportunity to recognize and respond to your own feelings. Your emotions are like mail that you send yourself to check in with how you're doing. They play a huge role in sensation by recruiting the body's neurotransmitters and hormones, just like physical sensations do. It wouldn't be wise to ignore when something hot or sharp touches the skin. In fact, our bodies are not programmed to disregard that information. Similarly, on the other side of the skin, it's not a great idea to try and block or toss out our feelings.

We all may feel pressured to suppress emotions on some level by family, friends, and society in general, but they don't really vanish when we're trying to disconnect from them. They hang around affecting our lives like mail that is piling up, crowding our space, and blocking us from moving forward. What is acne's biggest aim as a bully?

Blocking you from moving forward, living your life, and being who you are.

The unopened mail starts to gunk up our health eventually, which can naturally reach the skin, our largest organ of sensation and protection. Beyond the skin, suppressed emotions can affect how we see ourselves and discourage us from taking part in our own lives. We don't feel seen for who we are out in the world, and acne's trying to stop us from seeing ourselves as well. The bumps become everything, and acne tells us to be *nothing*. It tells us not to exist. This bully seeks to invade our skin and own it, which it has no right to do.

Feelings are a part of your life and only become a problem when they are told to shut up. Of course, we may get breakouts from situational or chronic stress, but this type of acne often resolves and heals faster. It will draw back when the stressful situation passes or when we take better care of ourselves in the face of daily stress. Acne tends to be most persistent and severe when there are emotions buried deep underneath. The bumps sit on the surface as an intimidating presence, perpetually trying to drive your emotions away from who you are. Acne doesn't care whether your feelings are so-called "bad" ones like anger and depression or "good" ones like happiness and excitement. It equally attacks all emotions that are naturally occurring human responses to life. When we are blocked from feeling, the skin is blocked from feeling too and its natural ability as a strong and vital boundary is weakened.

Emotions, including notoriously negative ones like anger, are actually protective of you and your skin. If someone mistreats you, one of the ways you can respond to protect yourself is by expressing the anger that arises. Similarly, if change is on the horizon, it would be difficult to prepare for it without some measure of excitement combined with anxiety. If you get a new job, graduate from school, or meet someone romantically, you may feel happiness combined with some fear of the uncertain future ahead. When you allow these feelings to exist and express themselves, regardless of the situation, you can shine through as who you are---both in your skin and your life. Without this necessary communication with yourself, you may feel as if you've lost your compass, and this is exactly what acne wants.

Acne is of course imitating any social influences that may be implying or telling us we're not allowed to feel anything. These messages can come from anywhere, but the most common dynamics I've heard patients talk about involve family. The people we are close to during our upbringings make a big impression on how we see ourselves, and the impact they make can have positive elements as well as challenging ones. The more suppressive and controlling dynamics that families experience tend to be born from the pressure to conform to societal norms and ideals, and this strain can show up in a few different ways.

Family members may think it's taboo to talk about their feelings, and this influence can change how we process our own range of emotions. We may feel unable to confide in our families, but also scared to admit to *ourselves* that we're going through anything. If we can't hide our emotions effectively, we may feel anxious that we'll get caught red-handed and punished for having them. We can then end up wearing a mask that makes us feel more hidden, not only around family, but around everyone—including ourselves.

The unresolved feelings in a family don't always present as uncomfortable silence alone. You may find that family members also have bouts of feeling excessively sorry for themselves, and they become intolerant of you not responding in the same way. There may also be an underlying feeling of hostility from suppressed anger that has built up within a family. Each of these environments can make us overly question who we are and feel paralyzed, rather than allowing us to naturally and healthily process our emotions.

Sometimes families may encourage a dynamic where everyone has to be happy and positive all the time, even around tense or strenuous situations. This pressure to be cheerful on the outside regardless of how you actually feel can make it difficult to experience real happiness and excitement that comes along in your life. Other times, an individual may be singled out in a family to accept blame and be the scapegoat for anything "bad" that happens, because the family won't allow their group image to be tainted by unfortunate circumstances. You may have experienced this role in your own life. The family's image gets to remain fun, breezy, and perfectly normal, as long as the fall guy is named within the group. When the family claims that this one person has all the problems, they get to bypass talking about difficult circumstances, acknowledging them as real, and handling them. But this shirking of accountability can come at the huge expense of health and safety in the family setting.

In each of these suppressive family dynamics, we feel like we're inherently doing something wrong simply by existing and expressing who we are. Oftentimes, these different patterns can overlap within one family. It's hard to admit when a family or other type of group dynamic is affecting us and holding us back from being ourselves. When acne breakouts occur, it's also easier to point the finger at everything else but the suppressed emotions. This may include gluten, mold, or even our favorite foods, for example. We need something to blame, because we may have been taught that denying feelings is not a bad thing and can't possibly impact our health in a negative way. We may have learned that it's the only way to be truly strong or confident.

True strength and confidence however, both skin-deep and inwardly, involve respecting and processing emotions. Our feelings are in fact our best allies when standing up to the four-letter word acne. It's important to know and sense that you're fed up with these pimples, and that they make you angry by interfering with your life. If you don't direct this anger toward acne and toward the social influences that resemble acne in your life, it gets turned onto you instead. Similarly, it's just as important to let in the feeling of excitement and to acknowledge what you have going for you that can bring happiness and contentment to your life. Denying any of these feelings puts us out of touch with ourselves and makes us more vulnerable to acne's bullying and its attempt to usurp our identities.

Acknowledging and expressing your emotions is an ongoing challenge, especially if you're not used to doing it. Acne creates an additional hurdle with a sneaky tactic it uses to try and keep you out of touch with yourself. Surprisingly, as acne bullies you, it also tries to act like your best friend. It assures you, hey you can rely on me, because I know what's best for you. The best way to feel, the best way to act, and the best way to live your life. I know what's best for your skin too. In facing acne, it is important to remember that acne doesn't have any good advice for you and is not your friend; *you* are.

Step six in facing acne: Be a friend to yourself and listen to what you have to say.

With yourself as a friend, you have a big and strong ally against acne. Acne may try to convince you to give up and feel nothing, but as long as you're talking to yourself as a friend, you can see acne's lies and bully tactics more easily. Feelings don't have to be taboo, and in fact with practice, you can recognize how important they are for communicating with yourself, your body, and your skin.

Instead of unresolved anger turning against you and your skin, it can instead be dealt with by your body as a normal and natural emotion. If you're feeling anxiety on a regular basis, your body can process that too as long as you're honest with yourself about what's going on. Maybe happiness or excitement feel forbidden because you've heard the message that you don't deserve to express them. Allowing your body to accept these feelings can help support the skin too. All emotions that you experience can get out of hand if ignored, just like anyone who's talking to someone else would get annoyed when being ignored.

Try taking a moment right now and simply asking yourself, "What's going on?" or "How are you?" Just like sitting across from a trusted friend at a coffee shop and catching up, the conversation you have with yourself can be laid back as you check in with how you're doing. If difficult emotions surface, such as anger, sadness, or anxiety, try not to label them and instead practice acknowledging them as they are. If excitement and appreciation for where you're at surface, you can enjoy this feeling. Let yourself look forward to life in areas that you're interested in. As you uncover unprocessed emotions, try and remember that your natural responses to life are not problems that need to be fixed. You may have heard messages from people in your life that suggest the opposite, but the truth is that hearing your own voice and what it has to say is beneficial for your health, skin, and life overall. Acne isn't directing this conversation, you are.

The more you become friends with your feelings, the less acne can use them against you as a bullying tactic. As you openly acknowledge emotions such as anger, anxiety, happiness, and excitement, acne will have a more difficult time using them to inflame, invade, attack, insult, or ostracize your skin. With renewed strength, your skin can better perform one of its major functions: Sensation. It can feel, not only the internal and external worlds on either side of it, but also itself. That's the true definition of feeling like you live in your own skin.

In summary, the skin is a living, breathing, and sensing surface, not just one that we put makeup and acne products on. It has two sides to it, and it likes to be treated well. In order for that to happen, we also have to treat ourselves well by acknowledging our own emotions and not giving in to the nothing, as acne urges us to do. Acne won't like it, but as you open your own mail, you reclaim the right to exist and to show your face in this world.

CHAPTER 6

You'll Never Be Perfect, But it's Fun Watching You Try

C ommercials that flash on T.V. for acne products can be cringe-worthy for someone dealing with chronic breakouts. A young man or woman washes their face with a sudsy cleanser and, after a few carefree splashes of water, emerges anew in the mirror with the most flawless skin you've ever seen. Do we want to believe that the product can do the same for us? Yes. But deep down, we don't feel like this miracle will ever happen and our pursuit for perfect skin will always be out of reach. These commercials are just sales pitches, but they are also symbolic of a feeling that people dealing with acne live with on a daily basis.

How many times a day do you think to yourself: "Why can't I just have perfect skin like everyone else?" Acne is a four-letter word that is clearly not perfect in its appearance, but it constantly makes us feel like we have to be perfect while we're wearing it on our skin. The distance between the acne we have and the perfect skin we want can seem impossible to travel. It makes us search endlessly for the magic solution that will change everything overnight, which ironically just keeps us feeling farther away from clear skin.

Acne is relentless in sparking or perpetuating a "be perfect" mindset, and it's not alone in its harassment. Even the skin care industry, that should be sensitive to how someone feels when they're dealing with breakouts, seems to plug the idea of overnight transformation and perfect skin. Doctors may imply that getting rid of acne is quickly achievable through a certain medication, or by eliminating gluten, dairy, meat, and sugar and eating the perfect diet. Estheticians often claim that the perfect skin care regimen will solve all problems of clogged pores and oily skin.

It's time to ask whether the chase for perfect skin perpetuates acne and feeds into its fuel as a bully. Acne constantly pushes you to aim for perfection, and the skin isn't the only area in which it's doing this. By shooting for flawless skin, we ask ourselves to live in an ideal way in which our health, lifestyle, and sense of self must also fit an expectation that always feels out of reach. It ends up being very unfair that we not only have to deal with breakouts, but we also have to live with so much pressure on our shoulders while acne is bullying us.

Acne's not just a bully; it's also a big hypocrite. In no way flawless, it still acts self-righteous and like it's better than you. Do you ever feel that? In the mirror, it appears like acne is red, angry, and trying to push you around, but it's also simultaneously saying: "You're nothing without me." Somehow, acne declares itself perfect compared to you and makes you work extra hard to live up to its "high status." Being a disrespectful presence in your life, this bully makes a lot of empty promises that you will eventually achieve perfection if you obey its orders, worship it, and keep trying too hard. In the background, however, it laughs while watching you shoot for a kind of ideal that is unrealistic and unattainable. Acne says: You'll never be perfect, but it sure is entertaining to watch you try.

People struggling with acne can be just as, if not more, affected by this pursuit of perfection as they are by the physical appearance of pimples. To offset the damage that this bully keeps inflicting on our skin and identity, we may try and act like we have it all together so we can somehow erase the feeling acne brings up for us. Acne is the real outsider on the skin and in our lives, and its presence feels rude, unappealing, and even gross. Yet, acne wants to hold a position of superiority over us and kick us out of what is rightfully ours. In order to maintain its rule over your skin, this four-letter word repeatedly insults you using these words:

I'm perfect, and you're actually the one who's ugly and gross.

Trying too hard to escape our flaws and the feeling of grossness that acne brings up is a hallmark of how people respond to pimples. If we can hide most everything except what appears perfect, we imagine that we're safer from acne and any bullying influences around us that mimic acne. We try and convince ourselves that by proactively plugging any holes of vulnerability, weakness, and insecurity we feel, that we can escape acne's insults and hide how much acne's really bothering us. We may even think that by being perfect, we can somehow trick our skin into being perfect too. So next, we get to work on making it happen.

Some people focus on making sure their public and social image is seamless. They want to feel perfectly liked and seen by others. This behavior can appear as going great lengths to please people, keep interaction on a surface level, and mask true feelings within social situations. Others will bring a headache-inducing level of perfection to their work or academic lives to cover up any weakness they feel from being around acne on a daily basis. You may try and be a model parent or homemaker, secretly hoping others will acknowledge the extra steps you're taking. For some people, it may be tempting to keep a perpetually spotless household because this seems to temporarily quiets acne's words. Maybe your handwriting is impeccable, your closet is labeled and organized inside-out, and you dread being even one second late to an appointment. You can drive yourself nuts trying to outdo yourself.

Like we've talked about, the need for perfection often extends into health and lifestyle factors too. Keeping the perfect diet, exercise routine, and skin care regimen can become an obsession to the point where any health potential from these efforts can get cancelled out. If something we eat contains even a shred of gluten, for example, we may drive ourselves toward extreme anxiety about impending breakouts.

It's also common to get entrenched in pristine skin care habits that trigger borderline panic if we don't follow them to a T. We may label all tasty and pleasurable foods as offensive because we're buying into the message that they directly cause acne.

These are all tendencies that, in and of themselves, don't have to be unhealthy, stifling, or extreme. When acne is driving you to overcompensate for a character blemish or deficiency it's labeling you with, however, all these habits ironically feed into this bully's agenda rather than keeping you safe from it. More than anything, an overly perfectionist outlook shifts the focus from taking care of yourself and your skin to instead looking and acting "right" all the time. Acne continues to drive the message home underneath the surface that no matter what you do, you'll never get where you want to go.

Acne's using mind tricks against you here, because being perfect is not necessarily where you ever wanted to go in the first place. Even before chronic pimples surface, many people are already exposed to the pressure to be perfect by family, school, social groups, or society in general (and most likely a combination of these). Just because people in general are bombarded by this message doesn't mean we don't feel conflicted about it. When acne comes along, it rides on the coattails of this common peer pressure and tries to declare that yes, you are in fact irreversibly deficient and flawed. It overinflates the existing pressure you may feel, and it claims that you have to try harder than anyone else to achieve perfection because of how far you've fallen from any ideal.

How does the pressure to be perfect affect the skin? It doesn't give the skin a chance to regain health naturally. This mindset can make people feel like acne is a very drastic, dramatic, and permanent problem that has no chance of getting better. While we're busy trying to be perfect, we also may think to ourselves: My skin is so far from being perfect that there's no use in trying. Acne then becomes a cemented stamp of imperfection that we're always fighting against, and the weapon we use to fight it is perfection—the very tool that acne's using against us!

All of a sudden, improving acne prone skin becomes an all-or-nothing health goal. It's tempting to want perfect skin, or if that's not possible, to stop caring altogether. Our efforts can start frustrating us much like yo-yo diets or stop-start exercise routines can. We're unsure of whether we want to back our skin unless it can give us perfect results in the end. If we expect the skin to transform overnight into a flawless image we have in our minds, then we're not able to appreciate any progress we make toward having fewer, less frequent, or less severe breakouts. We also can't be very supportive to our skin during the tough times when life is dishing out extra helpings of stress or challenges. The quest for not only perfect skin, but also a perfect life can be very brutal and self punishing.

Just like with anything else we want to change in life, the process and practice involved is still important when it comes to treating acne. If we want to set a more realistic bar for clearing acne that our skin can actually reach, it helps to first try and set a more realistic bar for ourselves as individuals. Acne may try and persuade you that having flaws and making mistakes is a horrible thing, and that being human in this way is just as heinous as having pimples on your face. That is actually a manipulative message that this four-letter word yells out to bully you and claim ownership over your skin. As long as you're not "perfect," acne declares that it has the right to torment you.

There's nothing wrong with having flaws in the first place, and that's not what is causing your acne. In fact, a perfect lifestyle doesn't exist out there that would eradicate acne from the planet. Apart from being influenced by hormones, diet, and other lifestyle factors, acne's largely a social symptom and bully. Have you ever noticed that acne can get worse around social interactions that feel stressful or that include people who don't see you for who you are? For that reason, acne becomes very intimidated when we stand up to any voices out there that are telling us to be perfect, act like we're beneath them, laugh at our flaws and mistakes, or ask us to follow a humiliating song and dance.

Step seven in facing acne: Learn to accept your flaws and challenges, and set your own bar for yourself.

By practicing this step, you show acne that it can't have control over you by setting your standards and telling you who to be. You tell it that you don't have to be perfect in order to have clearer skin, and that you're open to steps in the right direction rather than an overnight transformation into "someone new." Kicking acne out of your life isn't about being a new and improved person. Rather, it's about stepping back into your own skin.

Mainstream skin and health care may seem to imply that a perfect acne solution exists out there that leads to perfect results. Challenge yourself not to buy into that sales pitch, because perfect is both unrealistic and overrated. Instead, try starting right where you're at and allowing for the mindset that change can take place from this point forward. Not allowing yourself to feel good enough may sound like a convincing tactic coming from acne's mouth, but since acne's a straight up bully, we'll stand up to it instead and separate our voice from its voice. Trust your body and its underlying message to you that treating acne doesn't have to be an all-or-nothing approach.

Do you want to look and feel perfect, or do you want to look and feel like yourself?

CHAPTER 7

You're a Freak

---·---

A painful paradox about acne is that while it's on display for everyone to see, all you want to do as the person wearing it is *hide*. Sometimes you may feel like there's no place hidden enough to escape the world's sight and conceal your breakouts. It can be painful to imagine yourself as some sort of monster because of the way you look, and knowing that other people deal with acne too doesn't always help. You're not the only person experiencing this condition, but when you're being bullied by acne, it's common to feel very alone in what you're going through.

You may find that you especially want to block your face from those who know you well. Rather than sitting comfortably around a dinner table, kicking back at a party with friends, or trying out a new activity, you may end up gravitating toward a mirror or empty room to hang out with acne instead. It can be a relief to hide out from the potential scrutiny of others, and this disappearing act can almost feel therapeutic. The flip side of the coin, however, is that hiding doesn't make acne or your life change for the better. It can become a crutch that only perpetuates acne at the end of the day.

Hiding away can actually make acne worse. Wait—how can that be? It may seem counterintuitive to look at this connection at first.

After all, hiding may appear like the only safe option at times. It can be scary to expose your face, having very little or no control over how you look to others. The problem becomes that acne enjoys having you all to itself. It tries to sequester you in a little bubble where it can maintain control over your skin and your life. When you habitually choose to avoid everything "out there" in favor of worrying about your skin and attending to acne, you end up playing right into acne's hands.

There's no way to get fully involved in your life without being seen. Acne tries to convince you that being seen by others is a dangerous thing and that you could be attacked for it. It discourages you from taking risks and instead sells a "safe" life of anxiously staring into a mirror or sitting alone in your room, removed from everything. It suggests making yourself feel trapped. Does this type of life feel safe to you?

As usual, we want to replay the message acne is sending us so we can interpret what it's really trying to say. When we listen to the words more carefully, we hear the following: Go ahead and let life pass you by. No big deal. Hide out here with me instead, because I'm lonely and I need constant attention. No one wants to be around you anyway, because...

You're abnormal.

You're a freak.

You're the one who's repulsive to others because of who you are.

This bully is pulling you away from your life by using language that is very derogatory. In doing so, it's not just asking you to hide your face from the world. It's also encouraging you to hide from any unique challenges or obstacles that you may need to face in order to pave the way for clearer skin.

If you have a gut feeling that you're not your acne and that this four-letter word is the unsightly intruder—not you—then you're completely right. Acne is trying to push its characteristics on to you as a person, but that's not who you are. Having breakouts can naturally make you want to disappear at times and not show your face, but acne's extreme message that you're a freak because of what you're going through is just plain wrong.

When acne does have you to itself, it tends to make the following demand: Don't look away. It wants you to stay fixated on it instead of putting energy toward yourself as an individual. If acne were an actual person, you would even say that it doesn't want you to outshine it in any way. Why? Acne is a needy and lonely presence that doesn't want you to leave it behind. If you were to embrace your skin's natural attractiveness and your potential, you would see acne retreating in your rearview mirror as you pursue your life. These bumps on your face actually want you to stay and keep them company instead, and the more you do, the more fuel you add to their fire. Acne wants to be the center of your attention *all* the time, and the way that it's acting may be mimicking social influences that exist around you.

Is there an area of your life where you've been hesitant to be yourself, shine, or excel because you're scared of outshining others, or even a particular individual? It's worthwhile to explore the dynamics that may inspire acne to call you a freak and pressure you to hide. Acne often uses brute force to bully you on the surface of your skin, while the underlying messages that it's drawing from are usually more subtle and come from everyday experiences and social interactions. You may have become used to the attitude of certain family members, friends, or coworkers who seem content with you being overshadowed and held back by acne. Because these messages can get mixed up in the hustle and bustle of daily living, let's call them out and clearly hear what they sound like:

> *You're not allowed to be talented or show others what you can do.*
> *You're not supposed to be attractive or look better than me.*
> *I can't allow you to be liked by others or enjoy spending time with*
people.
> *You may think you look good today, but you're wrong.*
> *If you take any risks out there, you'll fail.*
> *I can see how incapable you really are.*
> *You're not smart or wise, and no one would ever take you seriously.*
> *No one wants to be your friend.*

Listen, there's nothing cool about you that's worthwhile for people to be around.

You're nothing without me, and if you try and leave me behind, things will go badly for you.

This is not your identity, but acne, and perhaps someone you know, is trying to label you this way. Rather than hide in a room, what you probably want to do deep down in response to this kind of treatment is get angry. Anger is a very natural response to getting bullied, even when someone's framing the mistreatment like it's for your own good, safety, or protection. The body is registering the anger, but sometimes we try and fight against it because acne suggests hiding is for our own benefit. These words of wisdom sound like a wolf in sheep's clothing, don't they?

We live in a world where it's not uncommon to run across people who are threatened by the unique qualities that make you shine as an individual. It's also not a surprise that these same people may use kind and caring words, just like acne does, to imply you should hide or sell yourself short. They may make it sound like you're better off being safe rather than seizing opportunities in your life and risking failure or humiliation out in the world. However, if you can't risk falling flat on your face or feeling embarrassed from time to time, you do risk missing out on rewards, success, or joy in your life. These "helping" words from acne and certain people you know may really be a disguise for their true intentions: to prevent you from outshining them or leaving them behind.

People may even imply that you're somehow being disloyal to them if you try and live your own life. Acne can take on this characteristic as well when you're trying to move toward clearer skin and a life that you desire. Often, people will find that when they take steps forward toward what they want in life, acne will strike their skin with a vengeance, retaliating against the change. It will make you feel like you're abandoning it when it's supposedly your ally and has your best interest in mind. Acne will even go so far as to imply that you can't live without it and you shouldn't risk leaving it behind, for fear of negative consequences. This bully is skilled at what it does and rather than keeping you safe, what acne is really doing is *holding you back*.

If acne is trying to keep us in a dark room, away from the lives we want to live, then the best way to stand up to it is to head out the door into the fresh air. Of course it's risky to pursue your own life, and to potentially outshine others who may not want you to go places for whatever reason. But the only thing that thrives in the dark is acne itself, not your skin or your life. Acne is the freak, not you.

Step eight in facing acne: Head out of the room you're tempted to hide in and see what happens next.

Preventing yourself from shining in your own life is not helping your skin get healthier. It only supports acne's agenda. You may at times think to yourself, hey—I can see my real skin underneath the breakouts, but it just feels inaccessible. I can't seem to reach it, because acne keeps blocking the way. You can start getting in better touch with your skin by allowing it to exist, and even shine for what it is. That means you let yourself be seen for who you are, even if it feels scary, risky, and you ruffle some feathers in the process. It also means that you don't label yourself as a freak and monster just because you're getting bullied by a four-letter word called acne. There is no more effective way to stand up to this bully than leaving the room it wants to confine you to.

If your life has felt stuck in one or more ways, then leaving this room is even more important. Acne has no interest in seeing you move forward through challenges you face or areas you'd like to grow in. Stuck is the name of the game that acne wants to play, and if it can keep you trapped feeling like a teenager in trouble forever, it will. This bully doesn't want us to grow up and gain confidence in ourselves as individuals, which is a journey that all teenagers must face eventually. Acne wants to shove you back toward feeling younger and more inexperienced rather than feeling grounded and confident of the steps you take in life.

Take those steps anyway, right past acne and toward the life you care about. The less you hide, the more opportunity you'll have to learn about yourself, your health, and what makes your skin feel right at home. Remember, anything that acne is trying to pressure you into doing is bad advice. Acne's voice can't be trusted. Though it may be tempting to stay home, fixate on one pimple, and fret about the best treatment, venturing out into your life will get you closer to clear skin than a "magic" zit zapper, supplement, miracle face wash, or gluten-free cookie ever could.

CHAPTER 8
This Is My Turf, Not Yours

---•---

Imagine the typical annoying bully who pretends to own the halls at school, steals your lunch money, and knocks the books out of your hands. He or she seems to linger around you constantly, showing up at inopportune times to harass you in the gym locker room, after school, or during a class break, for example. You're frustrated, because there are no clear boundaries between you and the bully and no space where you can feel safe and protected from this menacing presence. Anyone who has ever been in a situation like this knows that before being able to deal with this bully, you first must get sick of someone always taking what is yours. You have to start thinking: Hey, I should be able to walk down the halls too. It's my lunch money, not anyone else's. These are my books, and I don't want anyone messing with them. In the same way, acne invades your space and claims ownership over what is naturally yours. It basically wants your lunch money.

This four-letter word is first and foremost territorial over your skin. Even one or two pimples can easily feel like they dominate the complexion, and the rest of the skin doesn't end up feeling safe from future bullying either. But acne doesn't just stop there, as we've talked about. Along with taking over the skin, it can also feel like acne starts to seize your thoughts and your emotions. Then, this bully will try and have a say in what you should and shouldn't do, for example telling you to hide out in a room away from the world. It takes over and threatens what is yours, including your space, your skin, and your life.

You can imagine that in a school where a bully patrols the halls looking for you, this threat can easily get in the way of you doing well in your classes, socializing with other students, and enjoying the process of learning. You may even avoid joining extracurricular activities or staying late for a tutoring session, aiming to escape the school environment as much as possible. Your mind is on what this bully will do next, instead of on what you want out of school. Acne similarly follows you everywhere, coloring everything you do and often making it impossible to have a clear mind toward your life.

Acne doesn't respect the skin's natural boundary, nor does it respect your boundaries in general. As an individual, it's natural to want things for yourself, but acne is a bully that is very much against that idea. It knows what you want, it knows what you already have going for you, and it gets enraged. It puffs out its chest, glares at you, recruits its nasty friends, and declares:

This is my turf, not yours.

It claims ownership. It says: No boundaries. What does life look like without boundaries? On the skin, it can lead to chronic acne, but this dynamic can extend into all areas of life when it's present. It can feel like an invasion of privacy and your space. It can allow people to assume the right to take what is yours. Without social boundaries, your road to getting what you want can get rockier and more stressful than it has to be. Even if you do get what you want, unclear or absent boundaries can make those things feel in danger somehow. It's as if external circumstances can come along at any time and snatch what is yours, much like the hallway bully. Acne plays this type of role on your skin, but it's likely imitating social dynamics that have already been blurring your boundaries and trespassing on your space and your health.

When someone—or something in the case of acne—keeps trespassing on what is naturally your turf, it makes sense you'd want to fight back. With acne, too often we turn toward strongly medicated treatments, harsh products, and picking at our pimples as a means to go to war. When we are taking this route, we actually end up attacking the skin itself more than we end up making a dent with acne's invasion. We may also end up attacking ourselves mentally and emotionally, frustrated that our head-on efforts keep making us and our skin feel worse.

Acne retaliates to this combative approach. It's already better at it than we are, and it will keep expertly charging back at us, often with more force. People who start and later stop pharmaceutical acne treatments are usually familiar with this outcome. When effective, strong medication can make it seem like acne has been driven away for good. Acne has no choice sometimes but to bend to chemicals that are in these treatments. When the treatment stops, however, it is common for acne to return with a vengeance.

While we do want to protect our turf from this four-letter word, we don't want to do it in a way that also harms us and our skin. Unfortunately, the skin care and health care industries are riddled with ways to attack our skin in this manner. Because acne is often seen simply as an excess of bacteria and an imbalance of oil on the skin, we tend to target both with potentially harsh products. These types of treatments can strip the skin of its natural layer of hydration, immunity, and vitality. In the process, they may wipe away acne in a similar way to scorching a field, but the feeling of invasion continues as we go to war with our own skin.

You need space, both from acne and from invasive influences in your life. Stepping back from a head-on battle can help carve out that space and allow for growth and health to occur. Acne constantly wants to remind you that even when you're not dealing with it, it's still around every corner waiting to snatch away your lunch money. Sure, it can and probably will pop out of nowhere to harass and threaten you. But how you deal with its claims of "ownership" over your skin, both when you're near it and away from it, determines how much power this bully can exert over your life. If you believe its declaration, acne can become your life, and vice versa. If you remember that your skin and your life are your domain, then even though challenges can come up to test their boundaries, you can recognize acne for the unwelcome intruder it is and reclaim your turf.

Step nine in facing acne: Walk the halls, because it's your right.

The only way to protect your turf is to live there. Acne may come along, and when it does it will certainly affect you, but it doesn't have to own you. If you're always looking over your shoulder to see where this bully is standing and when it might appear next, it becomes more difficult to live your life and ironically, to protect the boundary of your skin. Your eyes are on acne, not on the things that can naturally strengthen, nourish, and support your skin. This hypervigilance plays into acne's wicked strategy, and while your boundaries are unprotected, it will have a heyday invading your skin.

People who walk all over your boundaries in everyday life can also affect your skin, even though as a society we don't openly talk about this connection. It's up to the individual to decide where their boundaries lie, what types of behavior cross the line, and how to make boundaries clear around people. We're encouraged from a young age into adulthood to please others, and this tendency can make it challenging to confidently express boundaries when we need them the most. We may feel concerned about displeasing those we know in the process of standing up for ourselves, and so instead of honoring our own limits, we end up doing nothing when we feel mistreated.

How does it affect your health when you're pleasing everyone except yourself? Basically, it's like taking the lunch money out of your pocket and just handing it out instead of risking facing and standing up to the bully in the hallway. It can get to the point where not only are people overstepping your boundaries, but you also start doing it to yourself, encouraging a domino effect where your limits no longer matter. You say: Hey everyone, here's my lunch money! Come and get it!

Don't surrender your turf just because it may seem easier or simpler in the moment. Moments stack on top of one another, and eventually as boundaries get increasingly blurred, the stress of influences invading your turf can affect the skin and your life overall. When you make your boundaries known, you may feel some guilt or fear of displeasing others, and some people who've come to expect you to be a certain way may get angry at you for it, but you also invite healthier interactions into your life for the long-term. Healthier social interactions can help protect your turf against bullies like acne.

If you're not sure what your boundaries are, ask yourself what you want. If you see that certain obstacles keep standing in the way of what you want—whether it's clear skin or anything else in life—then those road blocks often point the way to vulnerable areas of your turf. You can then ask yourself: How do I strengthen and support that space so I can move toward what I want? These questions naturally point you to boundaries that you can put in place for yourself.

As our world has become less private, interconnected with technology and geared toward social media followers and over-sharing, it's more important than ever to recognize your own turf and support the health of it. Greater connection among people doesn't necessarily always support the connection we have with ourselves; in fact, sometimes it's the opposite. It can be easier to feel a disconnection from yourself and your turf in today's modern social environment.

It's your lunch money, your skin, and your life. A four-letter word like acne doesn't own your space, and neither does anyone else. It turns out that yet again, acne is wrong. *Your skin is your turf, not acne's.* Supporting the skin's boundaries by strengthening yours will help you stand up to this bully for the long-term. Remember, acne may act all tough and commanding on the outside, but it's a coward at heart just like any bully is. The more you own your presence and connect with your turf, the more acne reveals itself as the puny bully that it is.

CHAPTER 9

How People See You Is All That Matters

———— • ————

Those dealing with acne may care a lot about how others see them, and the breakouts seem completely to blame for this. It's easy to think that if our skin were perfect, then we wouldn't focus as much on what others think about us. Is this necessarily true? We've reached yet another chicken or egg question:

Did acne make us overly concerned with how others see us, or were we already feeling that way before acne came along? Acne is an opportunistic bully, and it tends to strike most where we're already feeling exposed or vulnerable. Focusing on what others think is a challenge everyone faces in their lives, but for people dealing with acne, this struggle becomes visible on the skin and affects appearance. As much as we don't want acne around, it bullies us so relentlessly that we come face-to-face with any fears about how others see us and how we see ourselves.

Doctors don't typically pull out their clipboards and ask:

On a scale of 1 to 10, how much do you allow other people's opinions of you to affect how you see yourself?

Even though this question doesn't come up, fixating on what others see places a wrench in how we treat ourselves and take care of our bodies. Instead of turning inward and asking what the body needs during tough times, we risk caring more about how we look to everyone else. We may inadvertently neglect or reject what is good for us so we can be approved of by others and not appear un-cool or stupid. We may even fear that by doing what is best for us, we'll stand out in a group and no longer fit in.

You don't need a lab test or physical exam to confirm how awful it can feel when your image takes priority over how you see yourself. For many people, this conundrum also makes their skin look and feel worse. While acne is urging you to stare at your flaws, blemishes, and imperfections, it reinforces a bullying message that is often already in place. This message states that other people have a right to nitpick your identity, to point out everything that's wrong with you, and to proclaim that they know you better than you know yourself. When acne dominates your skin, the situation can even feel familiar and comfortable, because it may match how you're already feeling.

Monitoring what others think of you may appear like a wise decision in the moment. No one likes being seen in a light that doesn't match who they are. However, if you dedicate too much time trying to create a flawless image for others to see, you may increasingly live outside of your skin and shift into a world where you're seeking approval—mentally and energetically, as well as physically. Over time, you may see yourself more through the eyes of others than through your own eyes.

Acne will tell you this is the right direction to follow. Remember—you don't want to trust acne, because it's a bully. The key to standing up to it doesn't involve spending all your time wondering how others see you during a breakout. This only perpetuates the problem. It's natural to feel self-conscious with acne on your skin, but this feeling doesn't have to become a statement of who you are as a person. Typically, those with acne wonder not only how people see their skin, but also how others are scrutinizing their personality, actions, and life overall.

The nitpicking of your skin and who you are as a person can continue for the long-term, if you let it. This habit will never let you feel satisfied that you "look right," regardless of what your skin looks like. Eventually, what you imagine others might be thinking about you can start to become your reality. This way of thinking tends to assume the worst and doesn't give you credit for anything that makes you who you are. If you get used to picking apart everything about you, acne will give you a never-ending source of material to work with.

As a human being, it will be natural that you'll wonder what others think about you, especially when your skin isn't in the condition you wish it were. But you can still stand up to the declaration acne keeps hammering at you:

How people see you is all that matters.

Acne is wrong. How people see you is a part of life, because everyone has eyes and can form an opinion of their own. Sometimes people may use what they see constructively, to support you, guide you, and promote health. Other times, however, opinions can be used as a means to suppress, control, and even slander you. There are people who may "see" you in this way in order to have power over you, or to project feelings about themselves onto you. When sight is used in this way, it can naturally have a detrimental effect on the skin, which is the first part of us that people see.

There is no magic force field that can block our awareness of what other people may be thinking, feeling, or saying about us. What we can do, however, is minimize prioritizing this view over our own, as well as question some people's motives for their critical views. When you see yourself clearly and feel that others are labeling you in an unfair way, you can still keep your own view of yourself alive and active in your life. You don't have to look toward others to see yourself. If you're serious about kicking acne to the curb and experiencing clearer skin, others won't provide the spark to get there. You'll ignite the spark by seeing yourself for who you are.

Step ten in facing acne: See yourself through your own eyes.

It's natural to want others to reflect that they see the real you, and some people will, but not everyone. We can end up disappointed when instead of getting seen and supported for who we are, we get labeled, insulted, or misrepresented in return. When this does happen, it helps to be honest about the dynamic that's taking place. Quite often, we don't want to admit that what others think about us might be affecting us. Our society, while it habitually watches and scrutinizes people, loves to simultaneously urge us "never to care what others think." That's a catch-22 that creates a lot of stress and confusion, and it tends to undermine us when we're trying to be real about our experiences. The truth is, there is no cloak of immunity from these dynamics, but what people are saying or thinking about you doesn't have to take over your life and who you are.

When we can't admit how we're being affected by these opinions in the first place, we risk letting them insidiously seep into our skin and life. They quietly make themselves right at home, and inadvertently we let them negate what really matters. We think that by ignoring them, they'll go away on their own. You may even hear the common message out there to "just be yourself" from T.V. shows, commercials, media, music, culture, and society overall. They make it sound like a walk in the park, something that you just absorb from breathing without any effort. But in real life, we innately know that you have to fight to have the courage to be in your skin. Unlike advertised, you can't do it in a vacuum where the challenges we've talked about don't exist.

It may not always feel fair to have to deal with the pressures of how others see you. The labeling doesn't stop, and peering eyes are always around when you least want them to be. It can be unsettling to face this reality. We often imagine that if we spend time trying to solve the problem of how others see us, that we'll eventually be standing on the other side of this dilemma. We'll never have to deal with it again, be affected by it, or be slowed down by what others say about us. Then we'll have perfect skin and acne will no longer have power over us.

The truth is, there is no solution. The more we try and fix these faceless messages, the more we end up trying to fix ourselves. In the face of acne and other bullies like it, we need the confidence to know that we don't need fixing, regardless of what others say. You can allow your strength of character to support you instead of waiting for others to approve of what they see. That means you may not always feel normal around other people, especially those who are judgmental toward you. But maybe being normal to others isn't what matters most. Your skin is naturally strengthened when you stay connected to yourself through your own eyes, regardless of what others see.

Acne is a bully that will always urge you to reduce yourself to a walking zit for others to glare at. It suggests that everything "wrong" with you, such as imperfections and weaknesses, should lead the way. It seeks to label you using what others may judge on the outside. And it torments your skin, in the pursuit of making people see the worst. However, you don't have to sit by and take it. Acne has no idea how much power you possess against its tactics just by keeping your eyes open about who you are. You'll naturally see faults and weaknesses because you're human, but you'll also notice your strengths, uniqueness, courage, and attractiveness.

When you dig deep and look at yourself clearly, it's not just clear skin you're promoting in the face of acne. You're also empowering your life with energy that would otherwise be wasted comparing yourself to the image others see. Sure, it'll affect you from time to time that people can be critical and unfair, but you'll also have more energy to face these feelings and not get stuck in the judgment. You'll show acne that its influence is ultimately shallow, because the core of who you are isn't just skin-deep. Allowing yourself to radiate as an individual regardless of what others say about you is the best elixir for your skin, both in and out.

CHAPTER 10
Just Give Up Already

Y̲ou know the feeling when you've just gotten over one annoying pimple or breakout, and then another one pops up almost immediately? You haven't even had a chance to enjoy getting rid of one acne flare-up when another one surfaces to bully you more. This seemingly never-ending cycle can be exhausting. The truth is, acne wants to wear you out over time.

The scariest thing about bullies is the implication that they're never going to stop. Their behavior shows no intention of making peace, calming down, or being reasonable. Instead, they tend to ramp up their mistreatment of you during the worst times. For example, when you're feeling stressed, overwhelmed, or tired, that is when acne tends to rear its head the most. During times you're trying to ace an exam or achieve something, acne will try and block the way as a distraction. When you want to look good for a social event, presentation, or job interview, acne will stand up, wave, and say, "Not today." In that sense, acne is very opportunistic.

Over time, things like acing an exam, achieving what you want, looking good, and being present at a social event can start to feel impossible. The interests that you'd like to put time and energy toward may seem out of bounds as long as acne's around. You may wonder:

How did one physical symptom—a zit—start to stand in the way of everything you care about?

Acne doesn't want you to care about anything other than it. As we've talked about, this bully actually goes so far as to label you as a freak, loser, and as someone who's gross in order to trap you in its world. If acne were to have its way, this trap is supposed to get stronger over time. Eventually, you're supposed to barely be able to see past it. Acne's ultimate message is:

Just give up already.

Many of us with acne don't want to face this underlying feeling that comes up. We may try extra hard to show that we're motivated, ambitious, and hard working to counteract acne's bullying and the pressure it puts on us to stop caring. But no matter what we do, it never feels like enough. The "give up" feeling can resurface along with acne every time a new breakout occurs and make it challenging to build real momentum toward the things you want.

Eventually, you may find that you don't want to deal with anything. But it's not your life you don't want to deal with anymore—it's acne. The two can easily get confused, and because the mentality can develop that acne is permanent and there's no chance of confronting its incessant bullying, we may give up on ourselves instead.

Acne pressures us to give up on our health along with everything else. Our skin then becomes a disappointment, a symbol of something that failed us and didn't stick up for us in the face of acne. What we often miss in that moment is that first we have to stick up for ourselves, not just around acne, but around anyone who wants to disrespect us. If someone is treating you like you're nothing, unworthy, a freak, a disappointment, a failure, or a loser, that's all connected to your skin and acne's invasion of it. Until you stand up to those influences, the skin remains vulnerable to a bully like acne.

You want a life you can call your own, and that's not a crime. Wanting to live and experience life can actually start to feel impossible in the presence of acne. It can also feel futile around social influences who keep urging you to hold yourself back from your potential and what you're capable of. Acne is very tied in to the hopelessness we may feel about having our own lives in general.

Throughout this book, we've been covering various steps you can take to face acne. Here is one more very important one to add to the list:

Step eleven in facing acne: Don't give up.

It can feel so tempting at times to give up on your skin and other areas of your life that are affected by acne. Especially when treatments or products aren't working, someone is staring at your skin, or you have to look at your breakouts in photos, you may want to throw in the towel to this bully. Acne just seems so strong, and at times we become convinced that it's stronger than us.

You're stronger than it. Don't give up on your skin, because whether you can see it or not, your skin has the potential to stand up to acne. You do too. Giving up may offer a lifetime membership of hiding behind acne and feeling "safe" behind this bully, but the reason you're reading this book is probably because you don't want that.

Refusing to give up doesn't mean you have to run out and purchase new acne products, turn your diet into the typical menu of a squirrel, or visit every doctor, healer, and esthetician out there. You don't have to try that hard to force acne away. Instead, you can start your unique journey of facing the real life challenges that are behind acne's presence, standing up to these zits, getting used to the idea that you deserve attractive skin, and allowing yourself to exist for who you are. Basically, you're making this four-letter word a lot less important, and making yourself matter most in your life.

Acne's not going to shut up on its own, and it doesn't care very much about the efforts we take to appease it. You can buy the most expensive skin care product out there, and this bully may still bulldoze over your purchase to create more breakouts. You can eliminate all dairy, gluten, and sugar and find that acne laughs at you for trying to change your diet. What can make acne shut up? When you don't play nice with it anymore. You show it that it's just another stupid four-letter word and nothing more.

We've now talked about the real face of acne, how to recognize the curse words that it uses against us, and steps we can take to stand up to this bully. It's important to remember that your voice and identity exist separately from that of acne, no matter what it keeps whispering to you. It wants you to think you're exactly the same as it is, that your face matches acne's face. It also wants you to believe that it owns and has power over you without you having any say in the matter.

In the second half of this book, we'll talk about how to bring out your distinct, strong, and unmistakable voice in the face of acne's bullying. This four-letter word spends all day cursing at you, and now it's time for you to get a chance to talk back. What would you like to say? We'll build on the simple steps we've already covered and discuss some practical tools that can help support the health of your skin and let you reclaim it.

No more. Acne doesn't get to have the last word.

PART 2

SEPARATING YOUR VOICE FROM ACNE'S

CHAPTER 11
Choose Your Own Adventure

———————•———————

There are two completely different ways you can approach acne. Imagine one scenario in which fixing acne is all that matters to you. Everywhere you go, your actions are influenced by acne's hurtful presence, words, and accusations. You want immediate results, so you spend your time, energy, and money on finding the magic solution that will make the whole nightmare go away. The way you take care of yourself and your skin has a tortured and punishing feel about it, and underneath the surface, you honestly just want to avoid both your skin and yourself. The cure seems like an empty promise out there, so close yet so far away. While you're busy blaming yourself for your skin, you're also trying to create impossibly perfect circumstances in your life surrounding diet, skin care, health, thoughts, and emotions.

Many of us who have experienced chronic breakouts are already familiar with this first scenario. It creates a cyclical pattern of acne, bullying, and guilt about who we are. Each time we try something new for our skin, we sigh, feeling discouraged about the outcome we imagine will occur. More bullying from acne. Nothing becomes possible using this approach and acne gets to be (annoyingly) right all the time. It's a defeating experience.

Now picture a different scenario: You decide that that you won't take bullying from acne any longer. You're sick and tired of this four-letter word creeping around everywhere with you, and you're sick of the guilt and self-blame it instigates. Acne is trying to intimidate you and make you feel fearful, and you don't want to live this way. Each time you face acne, you say no.

You may try various products or treatments for your skin, but your experimentation is no longer driven by panic, superstition, and desperation. It's a more relaxed "I'll give this a try" approach. Rather than facial creams or washes being the focus, it's your courage in the face of acne's bullying that leads the way. You feel more freed up to try new things and even allow them to be fun, including creative skin care routines or natural therapies when you're in the mood for them. Because your actions don't have to offer a solution or fix to acne, life can open up. You as a person finally get to stop revolving around acne.

In this scenario, you also let yourself see parallels between the bullying occurring on your skin and any suppressive, belittling, or disrespectful social influences in your life. You decide to say no to these dynamics as well, because they can greatly affect skin health and add fuel to acne's fire. The effect of unhealthy social environments can take you out of your skin, and when you stand up to them, you can slowly readjust to being comfortable in your skin again. If you pick the second option, acne stops being a four-letter word that you can't talk back to. The courage involved in standing up to it can spread into other areas of life as well.

You're now at the fork of two vastly different roads that you can take in trying to clear up your skin, most likely with different outcomes and long-term effects. At first, it can be challenging to open up to the idea that you *have* a choice in how you approach acne's rude and belittling presence. Many of us with persistent acne will resign ourselves to the mentality that acne is in our lives for good, whether we like it or not. The concept of choice rarely enters the picture, especially because mainstream medicine and the skincare industry don't talk about acne from a mind-body perspective. Yet, most of us understand that the mindset we carry into other areas of life such as education, work, family life, business, and sports does matter in the long run. Chasing dreams using fear, self-punishment, and impatience toward a quick result will naturally feel different than pursuing them with the openness to learn along the way and the determination to back yourself in the face of any challenges that come up.

Step twelve in facing acne: Make the choice for how you want to approach your skin.

The first scenario we talked about may give you the impression that a magic cure is out there somewhere, and as long as you keep searching, you'll eventually find it. You may feel reassured that a quick or instant fix is possible, because that's what everyone in T.V. commercials, doctors' or estheticians' offices, or department stores seems to imply. This way of thinking assumes that there's a perfect way to look, feel, and live, and this perfection quickly becomes the pursuit more than the health of your skin. This choice also builds a life focused around acne, with each pimple determining failure versus success. It puts the bully—acne—in charge of everything.

Why look for the solution in the very thing that's causing the problem? If you choose the second scenario, you can still use products and acne treatments. However, you give your skin a better chance of recovering because you're directly standing up to acne's bullying influences instead of relying on external treatments to solve the problem superficially. You're making your skin care efforts and routines more effective as you work through the underlying roots of your acne symptoms. Finally, by handling the bully right in front of you, you spark the courage needed to stand up to suppressive influences that may be hampering life itself and stopping you from getting what you want in your health.

You might not have imagined that the real key to overcoming acne lies in you rather than an external solution. We often hear the opposite. If a quick fix truly exists, however, where is it? We run around in circles looking for this cure, but at the end of the day it might be more helpful to stop running and to make a choice about how we want to handle this oppressor. Choosing to stand up for who you are may not seem immediately powerful in the face of acne, but this action can lead to significant long-term benefits for your skin. When these improvements occur, they are often longer lasting than those brought about from common acne solutions.

When someone switches his or her mentality toward acne, it's not uncommon for products they unsuccessfully tried before to start working for the first time. There may be a face wash, moisturizer, or topical serum that seemed somewhat promising the first time that finally works after the underlying block to skin health is dealt with. Similarly, healthy choices surrounding sleep, diet, exercise, and relaxation practices can all get renewed energy and effectiveness from standing up to acne. Health and skin care goals that seemed impossible before can start to feel real and accessible, maybe for the first time.

The choice is between learning about yourself and your skin as you stand up to acne, versus searching for the ultimate cure that may or may not be out there. Acne is a four-letter word that tries to alienate you from who you are, so standing up to it can help you disconnect from this bully and become better friends with yourself. Reconnecting with yourself can naturally do wonders for the skin's strength, integrity, and health. Meanwhile, the search for a guaranteed cure may cover up some of the fear and insecurity that surrounds acne on a day-to-day basis, but it also keeps you closely tied to acne and somewhat reliant on this skin condition over time. You may even start to believe in a strange way that you need acne and wouldn't know what to do without it.

Acne and the "solution to acne" appear to be two sides of the same coin. They both feel fairly impossible to work with and often make people feel stuck right where they're at. It may be time to choose a different sort of adventure. Open up your medicine cabinet and look at what you've already tried so far. You can stick with the search you've been on, or try something new. Which direction will you go?

CHAPTER 12
Picture It

———————•———————

Have you tried to imagine yourself with clear skin before? If you close your eyes right now and wait a few moments, you can probably see it. Our imaginations naturally want to get involved in picturing acne-free skin, but we often dismiss what we visualize as just wishful, frivolous, and unrealistic thinking. As a society, we tend not to give much credit to this type of exercise and would quickly label it as "woo woo" before giving it a shot. What if it's not woo woo and actually has the power to spark your skin's underlying health and its strength in the face of bullies like acne?

Anyone who has played a sport, started a new business, taken an exam, started a family, drawn a picture, or done just about anything that presents a challenge knows that visualizing what you want is the first step to getting there. We wouldn't want to block ourselves from this important first step, because the picture in your mind helps spark the beginning of your journey. Seeing clearly what you want helps you commit to the process that it will take to get there.

Reclaiming your skin from acne is another challenge that is worthy of visualization. Acne is an unavoidable bully, because you see it in the mirror each time you look at your appearance. The constant image of ourselves with this skin condition can start to fill our minds and eventually make it difficult to see anything outside of that. Unfortunately, the longer you picture yourself this way, the more entrenched acne becomes in your life. Even though acne seeks to overtake your skin, that doesn't mean you have to envision your future with it. You can resist its movement by imagining your skin the way you'd like it to feel and look. There's no cost or risk involved, and it's a simple trick that I've seen work well for those with persistent acne.

The mind is a powerful, and often mismanaged tool in health and skin care. It can block our efforts toward getting healthy and instill us with fear, or it can work alongside our natural ability to support the health of the body. How you see your skin's future and your ability to stand up to acne can certainly affect the outcome you'll experience long-term.

Often, our experience with acne prompts us to label our skin and ourselves in a brutal way. We may stick with words such as ugly, gross, freakish, and impossible to describe what we're going through and imagine that this situation will continue forever. Insecurities will naturally come up in the face of acne, and it's okay to be honest about these when they do. However, you don't have to allow the discouraging words and the vision they create to defeat your efforts to clear up your skin. When the labels do surface, remember that it is acne's bullying that you're feeling discouraged about, not about who you are and the future of your skin's health.

You may not feel the potential right now for your skin to get better, especially on rough days, but it's there and more accessible than you may think. Your real skin is here, and to tap into it, you can bring it into as much clarity as you can using picturing exercises. Even while acne keeps urging you to see yourself in a harsh light, it's okay to see and feel your unique attractiveness. You may have to dig deep to recover this feeling if acne's been chronically bullying your skin, but it's worth it to get in touch with your appearance in this way.

Acne's telling you that it's a crime to look good? One of the first ways to belittle acne is to own your looks and what you like about them. We can easily lose sight of this connection the more we feel tormented by acne, and when this happens, acne tends to ramp up its bullying. Society's message about looks can also be confusing to deal with. On the one hand, it seems like looks are judged heavily in the media and throughout society's messages. On the other hand, we're told that looks don't matter and that it's what's on the inside that counts.

In reality, what's on the inside and outside are related to each other, and that is why acne can be such a frustrating bully to deal with. It's natural to want to look good, not just so that others notice you, but even more so that you can enjoy your unique qualities inside and out. The fact that acne can affect how we see ourselves and make us feel less attractive seems unfair. Again, it can be helpful to look at the chicken or egg question: Were there already challenges present before acne surfaced that made you downplay or reject your natural appearance? Some people may feel that it's forbidden to look good because they're scared of outshining someone who asks to get all the attention. Others may be in an environment that is discouraging toward enjoying attractiveness.

If you truly want to get your skin back from acne, that means you also want to reclaim your unique looks and attractiveness from underneath acne's chronic bullying. It's okay to be honest about this health goal, because it's not just superficial or frivolous. Feeling good about how you look often goes hand in hand with supporting the health of your body and mind. When people move from teenage years into adulthood, the transition presents an opportunity to appreciate the presence we have out in the world with our new independence. When acne comes along and starts bullying us about our appearance, whether during this transition or later on, women don't get to fully enjoy their unique feminine qualities and men are also held back from enjoying their masculinity. Acne literally tells you not to grow into who you are.

As you reclaim your skin from acne, you also get to own who you are as a man or woman. Acne doesn't get to tell you who you are or what you should look like. Feeling good about how you look is your right, and it's not one that acne should have control over. In order to remove the block that acne places between you and your appearance, it's helpful to explore how you've been judging your looks in the first place. When you're honest about how acne has colored your perspective, you start to make room for healthy changes in your skin. The skin you want is something that's innate and natural to your appearance, but acne holds you back from it with its relentless insults. Moving forward, it's about allowing what's already there to come out, rather than having to be someone different and forcing perfectly clear skin to appear.

How can you help your real skin to rise to the surface? Start by using simple picturing exercises that you can practice when relaxed or before bed. The act of picturing the integrity and clarity of your skin helps you own your appearance in a powerful way. Many of us think: How am I supposed to own and appreciate my looks while acne is still harassing me on a regular basis? I'll have to wait until acne goes away and my skin is clear before I can feel confident enough to own my looks.

Not true.

Like many challenges in life, the courage and determination to stand up to acne is something you benefit from owning now, even before you see any results. A basketball player can't wait until he has a high-scoring game or a win before deciding that it's worth it to practice playing ball. A business owner can't wait for a guarantee of success before she puts in the effort to create a quality business that may one day help her turn a profit. Waiting and hoping are two actions that acne loves, because in the meantime it makes itself more at home on your skin. In the real world, outside of acne's manipulative bubble, waiting and hoping doesn't lead to much.

Real results happen when you put the right kind of energy behind getting them, even while not knowing what the outcome will be. Picturing exercises can help you spark the energy needed to own your beauty, stand up to acne's bullying, and reconnect with the health of your skin. These exercises aren't about mind over body, but rather mind with body. Mainstream health care tends to cut this whole into half, overly focusing on either the physical aspects of chronic conditions or the mental aspects. In nature, there isn't meant to be an either/or, and one area isn't supposed to dominate over the other. When you practice the art of picturing your skin, you engage both the mind and body to work together in the face of acne, the way they're meant to.

The key to picturing is to have reasonable expectations while doing it, and to try and reconnect with *your* skin rather than some perfect idea of skin. It may be tempting to create a big fantasy around the ideal skin you desire, but then the vision would take you far away from reality. The more real the visualization feels, the more potential it has to affect your skin and fight back against acne. Perfect skin is probably not even what you want, if you think about it. What may be more satisfying in the long-run? The unique qualities of your skin and appearance shining through and reflecting who you are, rather than displaying the punishing effects of acne or other suppressive influences.

Step thirteen in facing acne: See your real skin.

Performing visualization for the skin is a simple habit to weave into your current lifestyle. It is easiest to do before bedtime when you're lying down, relaxed, and ready to sleep for the night. To enhance your body's involvement, you can try progressive muscle relaxation to help calm the nervous system before the visualization:

1. First, connect with your breath.
2. Then with each exhale, slowly release the tension in each muscle from head to toe.
3. Focus particularly on muscles that tend to hold tension throughout the day, including the neck, shoulders, upper back, arms, and chest.
4. Afterward, you may feel a slight tingling in your hands and feet, indicating increased blood flow and relaxation throughout your body.

When you're feeling connected with your breath and body, you can start to play around with images that embody change and health for your skin. For example, use your imagination to create cartoon characters and picture your skin courageously standing up to acne's bullying. Or, you can imagine that the internal and external environments next to your skin are infusing it with energy and vitality. Picture yourself walking down the street or looking in the mirror with skin that matches who you are. See the scene vividly as if in real life—you can even imagine the exact outfit you're wearing or a creative hairstyle.

The world that acne wants to create for you can often feel dirty, so as you close your eyes, try spending time in a place that gives you cleansing energy instead. Get away from nasty influences like acne or disrespectful people who parrot the same messages as acne. Try a sunny and soothing island with blue waves where you can relax and shrug off all your worries. Travel to waterfalls near lush greenery and mountains. Visit the moon, the stars, or some other distant point in outer space. Explore an underwater environment, where you can see exotic creatures or search for treasure. Any environment— whether real or imaginary—that makes you feel good creates distance between you and acne and helps you gain clarity inside out.

In a different vein, you can visualize the immune cells in your skin kicking acne's butt and sapping it of its overinflated power and bravado. Go ahead and picture acne as a mean and scared loser, one that you're separating your identity from. Is it "bad" to think of acne as a loser, or to hate it? Remember, acne has been treating you like a loser first, and it may continue to do so unless you see this bully for what it is.

Picturing exercises aren't only skin deep. As you do them, your feelings toward your skin and toward acne may surface along with the visualization. If they do, try not to block them, because they're important to the process. It's hard to remember at times, but having clear skin is not in your comfort zone yet. While you're engaging with your skin, emotions such as fear, anger, insecurity, and anxiety can surface, even though you're picturing good outcomes. Good doesn't mean easy. The more you embrace all parts of what you see, the more effective the exercise can be for your skin's health. At first, you may feel like the best approach is to just be "more positive" in how you see yourself. Instead, envision yourself living in your own skin and being able to appreciate the rewards of it. Rewards are often earned, so it's okay to feel a bit of a struggle come up during visualization and to see yourself overcoming it.

Whatever comes up, try not to judge yourself for it. The beauty of visualization exercises is that there's no right or wrong way to do them. You're the painter of your own canvas, and what you see through your own eyes is most meaningful. You can even extend beyond the canvas and picture changes for other areas of your life, especially ones that have felt impeded or stuck due to acne's presence. For example, imagine landing a new job or other opportunity that you've been hoping for. See yourself trying a new activity, writing, playing music, or enjoying any creative or energizing pursuit. As you feel yourself expanding your boundaries through your imagination, you are also expanding your skin's boundary to reach beyond acne's suppressive influence.

Maybe there are related symptoms that have piggybacked with acne in your health, such as digestive complaints, hormone imbalances, chronic fatigue, or weight gain. You can add these elements to your vision and imagine how they can improve as well. What can be deceiving about acne is that it draws all your attention toward it, sometimes eclipsing where else your body could use attention and rebalancing. Because the skin is connected to your body as a whole, attending to any other chronic symptoms you may be experiencing can actually improve the clarity of your skin too. In your mind's eye, see your body's systems working together to call out acne as an invader and kick it out of your life.

Here is another type of visualization exercise you can do right now: Close your eyes and take a few deep breaths. Now imagine a big screen. The screen is split down the middle, with the word "Yes" displayed on one side and the word "No" showing on the other. Now ask yourself whether you believe that your skin can be clear and rid of acne. You don't need to think about the answer to the question; just allow your vision to zoom in on the word that comes to your mind first. If you find the answer is "No," try one of the visualization exercises that we talked about and then recheck your answer to see whether it changes. If your mind still seems resistant to the possibility of clear skin in your life, try and explore any doubts that could be prompting "No" to repeatedly show up for you. Shifting your mindset can help free up blocks that you may have about your skin getting better and more resilient to forces like acne.

You deserve to enjoy how you look. Picturing helps you reconnect with the feeling you get when you *know* you look and feel good, regardless of who's around. You can call it looking attractive, cool, beautiful, handsome, confident, energized, or whatever you want. Acne's been trying to rob you of this important aspect of your life and at times it may feel like there's nothing you can do to stop this thief in its tracks. That's where visualization comes in. Looking good is not a faraway fantasy that's only accessible to "other" people, nor is it just a superficial thing disconnected from who you are and how you're feeling. It's a reality that you can tap into by seeing the truth: Your real skin exists right beneath the acne. By putting a face to your skin that helps separate it from a bully like acne, you can start shoving this four-letter word back—and out of your life.

CHAPTER 13
The Look Away Challenge

I t's time to face the facts: *Looking is not helping.* If you've been over-fixating on acne for a while and haven't noticed any improvement in your skin, a stare-down may not be the best strategy. We all do it at some point and it's tempting to continue, like an addiction. Like any addiction, the compulsion to keep going eventually becomes painful and can block progress toward having clear skin. Remember that no matter how powerful acne acts, it's just a vulgar four-letter bully that derives its energy from you. The more you look, the more energy and attention you give it. While acne's getting all the attention, who's not getting attention? *You.*

No one can make problems go away just by thinking about them constantly. When we put a magnifying glass to our pimples, critique them, and think about them nonstop, we may think we're addressing the problem when we're actually making it worse. It may seem like a harmless and neurotic habit, but it can become a crutch that ultimately keeps acne around. After a while, we come to expect breakouts and plan our lives around not only existing ones, but also those that may show up in the future.

There is an expression that goes "what you focus on expands." By focusing on acne, you expand its role in your life and invite it to do more harm. Without necessarily meaning to, you make it into a reality that is even larger than the breakout itself. You may find that pimples seem to grow and get worse the longer you look. This is not a trick of the mind; oftentimes acne flare-ups do get bigger and badder as we're fixating on them and waiting for them to go away. So why not look away? We may fear that when we look away, we're missing out on important clues that could point in the direction of a possible cure. More than anything though, it can be scary to look away because the habit feels protective. Our constant attention to acne creates the illusion that we can control it, or at least keep it at bay. By not fixating on our bully, we may feel more exposed and vulnerable at first.

When you spend your time focusing on acne, you actually develop a relationship with this bully that you don't enjoy or benefit from. This connection allows acne to feel more power over your life, and makes it act like a "boss" over you. Many of us treat acne like it's an authority figure, one that can get very angry and punishing unless we do what it says. However, acne's omnipotence is coming from us playing along with its power trip and not pushing back. When it comes to pushing back at acne, the most powerful tools you can use are often simple and underestimated. One of these is:

The power of rejection.

All along, acne has been striking first and trying to ostracize you. It rejects you on a regular basis and claims ownership over who you are. It tells you that no one likes you and that you don't belong in your own skin or anywhere else. Meanwhile, you're just supposed to sit back and accept its intrusive and insulting presence. If you're thinking that this sounds unfair, *you're right.* It turns out, you can actually flip the script and reject acne right back.

It's easy to overlook the power we possess to reject acne, because acne acts like it's better than us. By ostracizing us first, it ties us to it and creates a dynamic where we don't believe we have the right to fight back. It's like a person who declares himself or herself superior to you—in other words, a bully. We can get used to social dynamics in which we're supposed to be less than someone who declares the exclusive right to reject us. Oftentimes, after being rejected by a bully, we're not left alone to do what we want in our own lives. Instead, we're labeled with the scarlet letter "A" (for acne), and kept nearby so we can give the bully attention, approval, and energy. We're also supposed to tolerate mistreatment as the bully sees fit..

If you've been convinced up to now that acne's just a physically-rooted symptom and can't mimic the personality traits of an actual bully, think about how you feel when acne's hanging around you. You may feel like hiding and excluding yourself from activities. You may end up putting yourself down and labeling yourself as less worthy than others. You may feel like there's an intruder present who steals your thunder, and that they're entitled to do so. Remember, this isn't your voice. It's acne, acting very much like an actual person who is self-important and enjoys belittling you so they can look better in comparison. Why would we be obligated to indulge someone who acts like this? We aren't, but we often learn throughout life that it's easier and safer to let this type of influence have its way.

It's not easier or safer, and the battle we endure with acne shows us that. So it's curious that we don't hear more people talking about the power of rejection in healing acne. Mainstream healthcare conveniently places acne into the category of a purely physical condition, to many patients' detriment. Encouraging an individual to stand up to acne and to deal with the feelings behind it can't be bottled, encapsulated, or made into a cream. In other words, this powerful step can't be sold for high profits like anti-acne gimmicks or five-step skin care routines. Similarly, when a person realizes he or she needs to stand up to demeaning and disrespectful social influences in life, it can make a real impact on reducing acne and may cut down on, or even eliminate visits to the dermatologist's or esthetician's office. Healthcare providers don't really like that! Basically, no one tells us to reject acne because by encouraging us to stare and fixate on it instead, a lot of money can be made.

Here is what your doctor may not tell you: Acne is just a bunch of pimples that enjoy fronting as something more important than they really are, and they love it when you focus on them. Of course you'll feel affected by acne while it's around, but that's not a reason to give it even more attention and leeway in your life. If you're ready to try something new, take on: The Look Away Challenge.

The challenge is simple: When you're presented with an opportunity to stare at a zit, appease it with five different skin care products, or think about it incessantly—STOP. Instead, reject acne right there on the spot and move on with your day and life. You'll still be aware of the breakout, no doubt, especially when it's severe. However, you're making a statement to acne by taking away its spotlight in your life and by not indulging its "emotions." Acne wants you to feel down in the dumps along with it, but you'll be brushing past it and keeping your eyes forward on what's ahead and what you want to do.

Step fourteen in facing acne: Look away from the mirror and your pimples, focusing on the things you want in life instead.

You may be concerned at first that you're neglecting a problem that you should be dedicating your time to. There is no neglect happening here, and in fact you could say that plenty of neglect occurs in the minutes and eventually hours you can easily spend poring over the details of your breakouts. Acne wants you to be entranced by it, spellbound by it in a way that feels unbreakable. Meanwhile, many of us fall into the trap of ignoring our overall health, disconnecting from who we are, and obsessing on what we look like to others. The real problem is not the act of looking away, but rather the act of obsessively looking.

Here are some simple methods for rejecting acne that you can practice on a regular basis:

1. When you see pimples in the mirror, try the following instead of fixating on the acne: Step back, calmly continue to get ready for the day, and walk away.
2. Emphasis on *walk away.*

3. As you find yourself thinking about a breakout, try not to engage these thoughts and instead get active with whatever you're doing that day.

4. If your breakout is throbbing or hurting, take a few deep breaths and take a moment to de-stress and unwind, even if just for one minute.

5. When you have an acne flare-up that coincides with an important event like an interview, presentation, or party, tell your pimples that they're not invited.

6. Avoid indulging a pimple with tons of products, dietary restrictions, and rules. Instead, keep it simple and attend to the overall health of your skin, body, and mind.

7. Don't try and fix or solve it.

8. Rest. Acne is telling you to hit overdrive in your obsession over it. Ignore its commands and let yourself recover and relax.

9. Use makeup if you want, but don't go overboard. Makeup can't make acne go away, but it may lessen acne's presence and help you feel more comfortable in your skin if used in moderation.

10. Venture out into the world, keep your head up, and do what you want. Other people care less about your pimples than you think.

With these steps, you're crossing the line and saying "no more." That means you're not going to be an audience to acne's antics any longer. This four-letter word wants you to care about it *all the time*, and believe it or not, when acne notices that you're not constantly hot and bothered by its presence, it starts feeling useless. If you won't be a spectator, who will? When other people focus on your breakouts from time to time, that's not enough for acne. It wants you to notice and care the most.

Rejecting acne is one of the first steps in showing this bully that you're not going to be scared of it. It's not by any means a cure for this skin condition or a magic solution. But the more you practice this important skill, the less control acne can exert over your life. How? When you escape the bathroom mirror where acne is trying to corner you, you get to do other stuff! Fixating on acne takes up time and energy, which acne just feeds off of. We free up this energy when we take a step back from acne's obsession with us and proclaim that we're not obsessed with it back. Engaging with your life on a different level is supportive to the health and integrity of your skin, ultimately giving it natural protection against acne's stupid games. Most importantly, it takes the fuel away from acne's fire.

As you start this process, the mind may knock against your efforts and insist, "I can't move forward and do anything until acne disappears for good!" This fear-based message may tempt you to return to the bathroom to track acne's behavior in the mirror, making sure you don't lose sight of what it's doing. You may be temporarily drawn back into the vicious cycle of trying to predict acne's actions and pleading with this bully to show you mercy. If a setback happens, it's okay, because this is a practice you're developing and strengthening over time.

Just remind yourself to walk away again, and try to acknowledge how standing in front of the mirror and reasoning with acne only allows it to steal more time and energy from you. Acne's theft shifts what is valuable away from your life. You can help prevent this. Once you're out the door and on to something else other than acne's drama, it's easier to gain new perspective and see yourself as separate from acne. But as long as you're staring at the problem and wishing for an instant fix, you stop true change from happening for your skin. You become trapped in a bubble that acne has created for you, a small world where there isn't room for health, learning, or improvement.

You have two eyes, and you can choose where to focus them. Now is a good time to decide not to waste precious life focusing them on acne and its bullying behavior. Would you force yourself to watch a bad movie over and over again? Acne's influence is like a bad movie, always progressing toward a disappointing ending. The key is knowing in your gut that you don't deserve chronic disappointment from acne and that you can help decide where your plot goes next. By rejecting and challenging acne's authority over your life, you start becoming the hero or heroine of your movie rather than the victim. In this new movie, you stand up to the cowardly bully and work toward reclaiming your skin and your life. It will be a challenge, bringing up fears and anxieties at times, but it's a worthy one to face.

CHAPTER 14

Learning Where to Draw The Line

———————•———————

A s we've talked about, acne acts like a *person,* not just a skin condition. When we challenge acne's behavior, we face it like we would a bully who intends on standing in our way and harming us. The type of person that acne imitates is someone who doesn't acknowledge your existence or feelings, tramples all over your boundaries, and claims control over you. This person thinks they call the shots in your life and won't take "no" for an answer, even when saying "no" is the best and healthiest course of action for you. Does this person want you to connect with your potential and live a full and rewarding life? Not likely. There comes a time when standing up for yourself in the face of acne has to extend beyond your skin. You also have to venture out and stand up to people in your life who hold you back and treat you like acne does.

How can you sniff out the trail of people who are behaving in a zit-like manner toward you? There is one very important emotion that can help point the way. This particular emotion is one that suppressive and bullying people will tell you is very wrong to feel, much like acne tries to convey to you while sitting on the surface of your skin.

It's anger.

Anger has become an extremely maligned and exiled emotion in our culture and society, and yet when you look at its purpose, it's a feeling that is very protective of life. In nature, if an animal faces a threat and has to respond for its survival, it can't remain completely calm and mild as it faces potential conflict. Its fur stands on end or feathers become ruffled. Pupils dilate. Breathing and heart rate accelerate as the body becomes charged and prepared for any necessary action. Without this natural response, animals can't respond effectively to their environments and protect themselves when they need to.

Yet in human society, extending into our families and social spheres, anger is often looked down upon as an inferior and even dangerous emotion. Regardless of how we're being treated by others, we're encouraged to suppress anger and to feel bad about experiencing it in the first place. It's common to be labeled as a "certain type" of person when you are mad, and to be more or less excluded from those who are considered to be more happy and agreeable. It's as if everyone else has a golden ticket that makes them special enough to never feel anger, and you aren't lucky enough to be gifted with one.

If animals could talk and comment on the human behavior of outlawing anger, they would say that we're crazy. They would question how we can go about protecting our turf and our rights, standing up for ourselves, surviving in the wild (which our world is too), and keeping healthy without any anger. They wouldn't comprehend how we can distinguish friend from foe. They wouldn't understand the benefit of suppressing anger on a regular basis, or aiming to constantly please others and appear happy on the surface. Animals would actually consider *this type of behavior* as dangerous and a potential threat to ourselves and our environment.

The reason being, because it's false. Everyone as a human experiences anger, and trying to hide it or think it away doesn't make it disappear. Yet this is what we're all encouraged to do in order to fit in with others and society. We're made to feel guilty, bad, and even dirty for expressing justified anger and we're told to fix ourselves so that we can control our emotions better. Control often means eliminate. But you can't erase a real feeling, you can only drive it underground where it gets stuck and festers. The chronic frustration that arises from blocked anger causes some people to become irritable, temperamental, and even abusive. Many people develop intensified feelings of sadness or depression as a result of suppressing their anger. Society then tells us that it's "bad" to feel depression as well, and it suggests that we cover that up using pharmaceutical drugs, easily obtained from the doctor's office. It's an unfortunate cycle, because when we criminalize our anger, it is a sad situation that has repercussions on our health.

There is so much we miss out on when we banish anger from our lives. Number one is true protection from bullies such as acne or disrespectful people that come along in life. Number two is healthy change that can come about from processing anger and dealing with obstacles that are standing in the way of what you want. Number three is the full range of emotions in life, including happiness and excitement, which become less accessible if you don't deal with anger.

I doubt many dermatologists will tell you this important part of acne treatment, but you have to get back in touch with your anger if you want to change your skin. Anger isn't what is against you, it's bullying and suppressive influences that are, whether through acne, another person, a group, or societal pressures. At its core, anger born out of a desire to protect yourself is rooting for you to live your own life and to shine as who you are. Anger is closely tied to courage. The more you stuff away your anger to appease bullies and prevent them from getting mad at you, the more your natural and healthy response of anger turns on you and your skin. It becomes trapped and just has nowhere else to go.

Anger helps us establish our boundaries around other people, those who are close to us as well as those we barely know. It makes sense that as we block this emotion, the skin, which is our first and largest boundary, can get weakened and reactive. However, the way society tells us to label our anger adds insult to injury. One of the hardest experiences is to feel *guilt* for instinctively wanting to own who you are, protect your life, and stand up to those who are trying to stop you. When this happens, the tables inappropriately get turned. Those who are bullying you get to say that you are somehow hurting them. The guilt we feel becomes a constant warning bell in our minds that by standing up for ourselves, we are supposedly doing something wrong and harming others.

Here's a little secret: It's all a trick. You're not harming anyone with your desire to live, express who you are, use your potential, and look good. Bullies who, for whatever reason, want to hold you back are often skilled with the rhetoric to make you feel bad about all of this, but in reality they're just mad they can't get what they want from you. They're holding themselves back, and they often want to stunt your growth and health alongside their experience. Of course their language screams the opposite, so that you become convinced that you're doing something criminal by exerting your boundaries and valuing who you are. It's a bunch of lies at the end of the day, just as foul-mouthed as the four-letter word acne.

Step fifteen in facing acne: Don't shortchange yourself: Go ahead and get pissed.

Allowing yourself to get angry at any suppressive influence will demonstrate to you that you're hungry to reclaim your skin and your life from any bully, regardless of who they are. You won't listen to the insulting and derogatory messages, because you can see through these words and interpret the real meaning behind them. Anger gives you an x-ray vision that cuts through the B.S. that bullies use to try and control you and your mindset. It also helps you get in touch with your courage, which is needed to feel comfortable in your skin while surrounded by a world that doesn't typically root on individuality.

At first, it can be uncomfortable to invite the feeling of anger into your life, and you may have a natural fear of becoming a chronically "angry person." Maybe you tried to express anger in the past and were unfairly branded in this way by people you know, causing you to squash your anger instead of acknowledging it. It's suppressed anger that actually makes people feel frustrated all the time. Anger tends to naturally burn out or become less intense when you let it exist and deal with the threat that's prompting it. Just like with animals, allowing yourself to get angry in the face of a threat is what allows you to protect yourself and feel peace in your life.

As you're reconnecting with your anger, another important emotion may rise to the surface along with it—guilt. If it does, that's okay. It's important to deal with any feelings of guilt and remind yourself that you're not doing anything wrong by valuing your life. You have the right to own what is yours regardless of what anyone says, whether it's your personality, charisma, talents, looks, health, or unique way of relating to others. When you suspect that others are trying to make you feel guilty about who you are and what is special to you in your life, you can learn to recognize where this message is coming from and protect yourself from these influences. It's not your voice, but rather an external voice coming first from society and then, as an extension, possibly certain people you know well among family and friends. You can view your anger toward these influences as a supportive energy that's trying to free you from them, and guilt as the rope that tries to pull you back.

It can be alarming when you open your eyes and notice that people you care about are discouraging you from getting what you want in life. They may not even respect that you have your own life in the first place. The type of guilt that is pushed on to you by people who want to hold you back is different than natural guilt. When you do something you regret and genuinely wish to make a situation better for the future, guilt can come up in these circumstances and it can even be healthy. This type of guilt feels different and often gives you the opportunity to make changes that can help you learn from past mistakes and move forward. The guilt conveyed by bullies, however, is framed in a way that makes you feel there's no way out and no chance for resolution. If you don't keep your eyes open to what these bullies are doing, you can easily end up stuck in this type of guilt. Bullies love this.

People who are trying to hold you back in life may not be too happy as you open your eyes to their behavior. They might try and make you feel sorry for them as a way to get you further hooked into the dynamic. They may be fully aware that as you reconnect with anger about how you've been treated, that you won't be as easily swayed by their attempts at overstepping your boundaries. Oftentimes, people can use a mixture of blame, sentimentality, victimhood, and pity to keep you fixated on a social dynamic that isn't healthy for you and is creating an obstacle to growth in your life.

As we talked about earlier, you don't want to get fixated on acne because what you focus on can expand further into your life. Similarly, you don't want to get entrenched in social environments or relationships where you can't be who you are and express your boundaries. To create change toward better health, you may have to disconnect from what others want from you in order to stand up for yourself. You may have to risk displeasing certain people, being considered as selfish, and being labeled in unfair ways so that you can be there for yourself and your skin. Acne often imitates social influences around you that are belittling and disrespectful, so it's worth exploring whether you are dealing with people who are overstepping your boundaries on a regular basis.

So where do you start with this exploration? The first and most important step to establishing your boundaries in this world doesn't even involve other people. You have to treat yourself how you feel you deserve to be treated, and then you can create that standard in your social interactions as well. You might have to get fed up with belittling yourself, putting yourself last, and justifying others' mistreatment toward you. You may have to call yourself out on allowing others to trample on your boundaries and believing what they say about you. It will help to be honest if you've disrespected your own boundaries over time, providing a pass for others to do the same.

We don't ask to be mistreated by people or invite bullies into our lives willingly. But when these social influences do come along, we may inadvertently learn from them that our boundaries are not worth protecting and that we don't deserve to shine as individuals. Acne can conveniently slip into our lives right around this time, and we may increasingly get used to hiding our boundaries behind the condition as it claims control over our skin. When you put your foot down and decide that you're going to treat yourself better—with more respect, care, and grace—you hurl a double whammy against both acne and anyone who tries to tell you who you are.

Step sixteen in facing acne: Treat yourself how you want to be treated, and this practice will help you learn where to draw the line with others.

One of the ways you can treat yourself well is by giving yourself space. Acne, and social influences that are like it, frequently try and close in on your life and deprive you of privacy, sense of self, and independence. They're always watching, and by doing so they're warning you that you're in danger of doing something wrong. Then your own mind may start "watching" you in this unfair way, making you feel like you're never truly in your own skin and free to be yourself. You may think: I wish I could be left alone sometimes.

You have the power to give yourself space, without needing anyone's permission to do so. Social interaction can be a healthy, enriching, and rewarding part of life, but society by design tries to use it to displace the individual's part in his or her own life. There's no reason why the whole focus of life should revolve around other people. Attending to everyone else's happiness at the expense of one's own can contribute not only to relentless bullies such as acne, but also to a feeling of wasted potential and a life not fully lived.

As you give yourself more space in life, you can explore additional ways to treat yourself better like you deserve. If at first you feel guilty for treating yourself well, that's okay, just be patient and keep at it. Change always takes time, even healthy change. As you turn your attention toward yourself in a more caring way rather than primarily a judgmental way, don't be surprised if you feel a change in your skin, confidence, and desire to try new things. Slowly, people around you will also learn what you expect in regards to how you want to be treated. As your boundaries become reinforced and people don't get a free pass to tread all over them, acne will start losing momentum too. It will have fewer people to imitate when it's trying to bully your skin.

You may find that not all relationships stay the same as you demand respect and better treatment. People you know well tend to get used to you being a certain way, and sometimes a pattern can develop that's difficult to change. As you're getting healthier and more engaged with your own life, there may be people who will try and trigger fears in you toward the changes you're making. Change can already feel uncertain and shaky at times, and their guise of caring and "worrying" about you may only serve to heighten anxiety and make you feel like you're going in the wrong direction. When this happens, it's important to remember that you're in charge of your life and your decisions—it's not up to other people. You may not be able to keep all relationships intact and harmonious as you grow more respect for your boundaries, but the people who do stick around for you will be a healthier influence.

Dealing with any unresolved anger and learning where to draw the line with people will give you more space to be assertive in your life. Too often we think to ourselves, "I'd like to say 'no' to this person right now, but I don't feel like I'm allowed." In the back of our minds we may know what we want, but then feel unable to communicate the desire to anyone else. When we're battling with acne, we may be even less inclined to assert our preferences around others. It's as if having acne transports us to a teenage mentality, where everyone seems to know more than us and has the right to tell us what to do. How we assert ourselves in social interaction parallels how we handle acne in the long run. Standing up to acne involves saying "no" and deciding what you want to focus on outside of this bully. The same goes for interacting with people—you have to be able to say "no" when needed, and to be upfront about who you are and what you want.

The skin can reflect to us how we're being treated by others and whether we're allowing people to overstep our boundaries. Though it's not the easiest dynamic to look at, taking on that challenge allows you to explore the root of the problem. The root of acne doesn't spring from using the wrong face wash, eating gluten occasionally, or touching your face. It also doesn't exclusively arise from hormone imbalance, digestive issues, or vitamin deficiencies. The underlying source of acne is often a lot simpler than that, and it can often point to challenges that you've faced while trying to navigate the social world around you. As you learn to stand your own ground as the individual you are, you can strengthen your skin both in the face of acne and its human counterparts. Draw your line where you want and then challenge anyone, or anything (in the case of acne), to overstep it— you'll be ready.

CHAPTER 15
It Won't Take a Miracle

—————— • ——————

For many who deal with chronic acne, waiting for it to go away is like wishing for a winning lottery ticket. We've been instilled with the idea that stopping acne is just one step away—but it happens to be a huge step that is supposedly based on luck and a wild goose chase. The feeling of buying a lottery ticket may be exciting at first, but it also comes with a sense of hopelessness. Especially as you purchase more tickets and see them yield nothing in return, the excitement starts to plummet and a sinking feeling enters that you're wasting your time and money. I'm not saying you shouldn't buy a lottery ticket, but approaching acne with the same "only one winner out of twenty million people" mentality doesn't usually work.

And yet many of us find ourselves there at some point. Our daily prayer starts to revolve around acne, with the same desperation of hoping for a winning lottery ticket. Enter: the quick fix. It's an idea that mainstream healthcare loves to push, even toward a chronic and persistent skin condition such as acne. They know that we're hoping for a lottery win, and they claim they can offer it. Worse than the many useless treatments and products we purchase and later toss out is the insidious belief that creeps into our lives. We start to think that clearing up our skin will be nothing short of a miracle. We travel a road filled with both doubt and reverence, thinking that a magic solution will appear one day, inside a jar of cream, tube of ointment, or bottle of pills. We may have a gut feeling all along, however, that the experts don't have a clue, much less a cure. They seem unable to deliver the miracle, or quick fix, that they're promising.

At this point, many of us feel like giving up. If the experts can't solve it, we believe, then acne becomes just too big a problem for one individual to handle. Yet, the girls and guys we see in T.V. commercials for acne products seem to have stumbled on a miracle that makes acne vanish overnight. We wonder why that can't be us. Eventually, we won't accept anything short of a miracle for our skin. If quick fixes are being promised, then that's the only feasible option out there. We develop a miracle mindset, waiting endlessly for an outcome that we've already determined is near impossible.

A lot gets put on hold while we're waiting for this miracle. Though we may stay actively involved in the hunt for magic results from products, treatments, and diets, we often become more disconnected from our bodies and minds overall. We may quickly discredit any response from the body, even a "good" one, that doesn't resemble a miraculous overnight change. We may come to see our bodies and our skin as deficient and disappointing because they don't measure up to the perfect outcome we dream of. The value of real change goes out the window as the idea of instant, easy, and magical gets put on a pedestal.

It's a very alluring sales pitch we encounter, but the problem is that it doesn't help clear acne for the majority of people. I haven't met anyone yet who has experienced the miracle. And there's a good reason for this: Miracles by definition rarely happen, and an unexpected vanishing act of chronic acne would be very unlikely. The miracle turns out to be an empty promise at the end of the day, perpetrated by a society, and a health and skin care industry, that primarily want you to believe long enough to make a purchase. Do they care if the magic "solution" works for you? Regardless if it does or doesn't, they can rely on you to come back and try something else.

Now, as mentioned before, products and treatments can definitely serve as supportive and complementary tools on the journey toward healthier skin. They can function like a bridge, making it easier and smoother to travel from where you are to where you want to go. This type of experience is different than a miracle, because you are in the driver's seat as you stand up to acne rather than expecting a random skin care tool to do the job. The products being sold are not the problem so much as the false promise of the miracle cure.

The miracle mindset can appear innocent enough on the surface, but it tends to set us back more than we realize. It suggests that what is possible for others is out of reach to us. It lies by telling us that everyone else who has recovered from acne was somehow blessed with a miracle. It discredits what our bodies are going through while trying to stand up to acne and social influences that behave like it. It takes us further away from reality and from discovering the very real steps we can take toward clearer skin.

If you're imagining that it will take a miracle to get your skin back from acne, this feeling can start to spread to other areas of your life as well. You may come to believe that it will take a miracle to get a job, meet someone to date, be accepted into a degree program, pass a test, or achieve good overall health. Strangely, the more we wait for miracles to happen, the more unfair and hopeless life can feel. If the outcome is entirely out of our hands, then how can we have real involvement in our health and supporting the skin's integrity? We are encouraged to accept the reality of acne and to keep smothering it with creams, serums, and other tricks as we wait for something that we don't believe will ever happen. As our skin suffers, we can lose sight that anything desirable is possible in life without a miraculous intervention from outside us.

The next acne commercial you see on T.V. will tell you the opposite, but the truth is:

It won't take a miracle.

Though you may desperately wait for the clouds to part and an acne solution to fall into your lap, that won't have to happen in order for you to have clear skin. The acne-be-gone miracle is just an idea, one that is used to back tempting sales pitches for products, pharmaceuticals, and gimmicks that are meant to keep you hooked for the long-term. As much as we don't care to fight acne forever, who wants to rely on a product forever that just barely keeps pimples at bay? At our core, we desire to be rid of the harsh treatments, tricks, fads, and promise of miracles as much as we want to kick acne to the curb. Both acne and the advertised miracle of overnight acne-free skin feel oppressive in their own ways. When we keep hoping for a miracle, we're inadvertently inviting acne to stick around for the long haul.

The problem and the "instant fix" to it are just two sides of the same coin. They need each other to perpetuate the dynamic for the long-term. Often, when we purchase an acne product out of the hope for a miracle, it acquires an imaginary label of "acne supporter" in our minds. Rather than truly believing that this product will help materialize the miracle we desire, we start to see it as acne's accomplice. The frustration we feel after a so-called instant fix flops can be immense. Even if it does work to some extent, we typically wonder if the positive result will be long-lasting or eventually wear off. We can develop a toxic and stuck relationship with any quick fix strategy we use toward acne, whether it's topical facial products or overly restrictive diets, natural detoxification cleanses, supplements, or pharmaceuticals. These commonly touted solutions rarely help when we depend on them in this way, and instead they tend to further block our path toward healthier skin.

As we've been talking about, we need to take the focus of our lives off acne in order to reclaim our skin—but on the flip side it's equally important to wean ourselves off the miracle mindset. It can be difficult to realize that this approach is detrimental, because on the surface it looks nice and promises the things we want to hear. It claims to have all the answers, so that you don't have to go through anything challenging to get your skin back. It applauds all your efforts toward shopping for and devoting yourself to the instant fix, reassuring you that you're taking the steps needed to one day stumble on the right solution. The word "steps" is misleading though, because the miracle is only meant to involve *one step*. It's actually a gigantic leap from struggling with acne daily to never dealing with a single pimple ever again. If it sounds too good to be true, that's because it is.

Think back on other goals or outcomes that you've wanted to experience in your life, and that have come to fruition in some way. Most likely, your journey to get closer to what you wanted didn't involve one enormous step that placed you perfectly at the destination. You probably took one step to start out, and from there you gained some momentum toward taking another step. Your second step taught you more about which direction you wanted to go and helped you commit a little more to getting there and not giving up. You kept taking one step at a time with enough curiosity, openness, and determination to move forward despite challenges that came up. You probably had a lot of setbacks and detours too. Rather than the one-step wonder that a miracle promises, you found that successive steps put together helped you get from point A to point B.

It may be a letdown at first to recognize that acne isn't likely to magically disappear, but deep down it may also feel like a huge relief. In your gut, you may not have truly believed in the acne miracle anyway. More importantly, you'll now be able to connect with the reality that you don't need a miracle to help you achieve clearer skin. You can instead take *your steps*, one by one, toward standing up to acne in a real way.

Sometimes we rely on the miracle because we're scared of failing without it. We may not contemplate that it's possible to stand up on our own to the belligerent four-letter word, with all its demeaning and immature behavior. We may also not have quite done this in our own lives, by treating ourselves better and placing clear boundaries with the people around us. When you do see the "miracle" for what it is, which is a ruse, you'll realize that you had no real connection to it in the first place. The steps you take now toward acne can be ones that matter to you and that make sense in the framework of your overall life. You don't have to rely on weird rules that, up to now, haven't made sense to you. For example, you don't have to believe that chocolate is causing your acne if you haven't found real evidence of this connection.

Step seventeen in facing acne: Take steps forward that make sense to you, rather than waiting for a potential miracle to occur.

When you value your own footing over the "miracle," you start to notice any real progress you're making toward clearer skin, no matter how small at first. If you're at a very low point with acne and you expect a 180 degree change overnight, you would miss out on the little improvements that raise you a bit from rock bottom. It would be too miniscule for your mindset to register as important. When it comes to acne, observing even a little positive shift can make a difference, because it shows you that change is in fact possible. We become blind to that type of change when we're expecting a quick and complete overhaul of our present circumstances. Rather than using the small change as a springboard to keep going, we then end up back at square one every time a new pimple erupts.

Every little step you take toward standing up to acne adds up, and seldom do you go completely back to square one once your skin starts clearing up. There of course may be ups and downs and stressors that come along to challenge your skin, which happens to everyone. But the overall momentum of your skin's journey will lean toward health rather than acne, even when you encounter bumps in the road. If you carry through with the mentality that acne can't push you around anymore, and then you happen to experience a dramatic change in your skin, it won't be because of any miracle or instant fix—it will be because of you.

Relying on yourself gives you a better chance of succeeding in the face of acne, and it's actually the empty promise of a miracle that can make you feel like a failure when up against this bully. You can break this cycle for yourself. Then when you see the girl on T.V. with perfectly portrayed skin who is advertising acne cream, you can think to yourself: That's not real, but what I'm doing for myself and my skin is. It doesn't take a miracle after all.

CHAPTER 16

Let Yourself Be "Bad" Sometimes

———————•————————

Within acne's small world, being "bad" is defined as doing anything that you enjoy. This four-letter word keeps haunting you with the message that if you like something or are having a good time, you must somehow be making your skin worse because of it. Take a sip from a yummy Starbucks Frappuccino, and you're in danger of sprouting a new pimple. Try a new and fun makeup brand that isn't 100% organic, and you're jeopardizing the chance for your skin to get better. Savor a dairy-filled ice cream, eat some favorite chocolate, stay up an hour later watching a movie on T.V., experiment with a new and fragrant facial oil—it's all categorized as bad because acne has strict, arbitrary, and merciless rules for you. Everyone else can have fun and be "bad" sometimes, it says, but not you. Your aim should be to stay away from anything remotely fun, because you haven't figured out your skin problem yet.

Acne makes us walk through a metaphoric minefield, where we're never sure of our steps and always concerned about the worst outcomes. Yet, we don't always know why some things are considered "bad," and we don't always have enough positive outcomes to justify why we're abstaining from them. We enter a very limited lifestyle, as if we're sitting rigidly at a desk in school and getting gold stars taken away regardless of what we do. Acne never lets you really feel like you're being "good." Your default is always bad no matter what you do. It just won't leave you alone.

What acne doesn't tell you overtly, but shows you through its actions, is that whether you are "good" or not, it intends to keep disrespecting your skin. Keep trying to earn brownie points, it says, because it's the only shot you have. Acne doesn't keep its end of the bargain though by actually backing off from your skin once you're playing by its rules.

This bully labels everything you enjoy as dangerous, when in fact, it's not. Think about the messages we've talked about that acne promotes in your life. *You shouldn't risk going out into the world and showing your face. You are doing everything wrong. All that matters is how others see you. You're safer spending time with your pimples, fretting constantly about how much worse they'll get unless you stumble on a miracle cure. You don't know anything about yourself or your skin, so just listen to everyone else's advice, whether it works for you or not.* It's pretty evident when we hear the tone behind these messages that acne has no intention of steering you in the best direction for your skin. Could it be then that it's also wrong about what constitutes "bad" versus "good" in your life? It sounds like acne's just using these words to keep you trapped in its seemingly endless game.

You may already be feeling that Bad versus Good is not a fun game to play. In fact, you end up missing out on fun moments when you're overly tuned in to acne's definition of what's bad and good for you. The worst part is, most people don't have a lot of success in recovering from acne by playing this game. The game just creates more stress and anxiety on top of what we're already handling from chronic breakouts. More tension in our lives just creates more stressed out skin, which acne loves. So we have to wonder, why do we keep playing along?

Acne culture plays on a trend that we meet up with a lot in healthcare, society, and our lives—that of the yo-yo mindset. It's all or nothing. The whole idea of "practice moderation" when it comes to eating habits, exercise, and other lifestyle measures frequently turns into "stay away from nearly everything" these days. We are encouraged, for example, to stay away from carbohydrates and sugar completely. Abstain from dairy, for no particular reason at all for some people. Even fruit at times is labeled as being bad for health because of its sugar content. On the opposite end of the spectrum of what we *should* do, we get the impression that unless we're actively involved in CrossFit or visiting a gym five days a week, that it's not worth it to exercise. If we're not vegan, gluten-free, and eating a 100% organic whole foods diet, then we're not taking our health seriously and won't be able to eat healthy enough. The list of bad stuff we should eliminate quickly grows longer before we know it, while the list of what we're allowed to do gets shorter and shorter.

The elimination list typically includes things that are healthy and enjoyable in moderation, with minimal or no detrimental effect on your skin. The permitted list usually includes rules and regulations that are very popular in the mainstream. This list is very often made fashionable by some celebrity or other, whether it be from the entertainment industry or from widely recognized health gurus. There may be a few helpful nuggets here and there to take away from all this, but honestly, health care isn't so complicated that we need constant reminders of what to do and what not to do. Not many sources out there encourage moderation, and we're often told to blindly follow the trends around us.

That's when we can listen to the alarm bells in our heads that ask: Which idea or product is being sold within these fashionable health claims? We are being steered away from moderation because simply, extreme sells more. Implying to people that they're bad and that they can buy something to make themselves more "good" sells well, and it plays on the fear-based culture we live in. When you stand up to acne face to face, you come to the realization that acne's presence isn't born from a bunch of shortcomings in your health and lifestyle habits. You're not getting acne because you're somehow being bad all the time. Of course an overall healthy lifestyle can support your skin, but many people follow healthy lifestyles and still have persistent acne. It's helpful to read the hidden message behind the idea of "bad" when it comes to acne, because many of us struggle with feeling bad when we're getting breakouts.

Let's take a closer look at what's going on, and why bad isn't always bad. The yo-yo mindset of "bad" versus "good" is really a punishment mindset. You're supposed to make lifestyle changes under the threat that you're misbehaving if you do what you want. If you're living your life, being yourself, and enjoying new things, you're bad. BEWARE—this message is the same one that acne hammers on your head. The pressure to always be "good" and the solutions that go with it are opportunistic, in that they capitalize on the feeling of doing everything wrong that acne already promotes in your life.

Rather than offering any real solution, this pressure entangles you further in acne's problem-focused world, where you're constantly having to try and prove yourself against acne's declaration that you're inherently bad. Many people find that this mindset only adds more stress and anxiety to their daily lives, and it makes their skin worse rather than better. Standing up to acne should involve doling out less punishment on yourself, not more. Those of us who have struggled with acne tend to be hard on ourselves as it is, so we shouldn't keep following the voices that tell us to judge ourselves even more harshly.

You can practice independence from acne by savoring your chocolate without feeling guilty about it. Eat your favorite foods in moderation without feeling like a bad person. Experiment with makeup or skin care for your own enjoyment, without worrying about acne's response to it. Stay up late or sleep in once in a while if concerns about acne have been controlling your sleep schedule too much. Likewise, if you're just having a bad day, try not to always fix it. Acne often pressures us to make every day appear great and put together, but you don't have to prove to acne that you're perpetually happy and positive. Start questioning the bad list more and experiment with life in the way that you want.

As you go, you'll see that you can believe more in how your body responds rather than in what other people are doing and saying. A lot of what you hear about acne are just myths, stories that people go around telling each other. But now you have the secret knowledge that bad isn't always bad, and good isn't always good. Your skin will give you accurate information on whether something is actually "bad" for your skin. If it isn't, you can enjoy it in moderation and keep building confidence in your own decisions and actions.

Step eighteen in facing acne: Give yourself a healthy dose of "bad" from time to time.

If you do break out, try your best to resist the urge to reprimand yourself for "offending" or "wronging" acne. Trust me, it was going to show up anyway. You're just living your life and there's no reason to feel sorry about that, even if you get an extra pimple or two along the way. Unless you can see concrete evidence from your body that a food or cosmetic is making your skin much worse that it normally would be, there's no reason to overly restrict yourself.

Do you tend to restrict your experience in areas outside of health and lifestyle as well? Perhaps acne has been suggesting that you'd be bad if you enjoyed a certain activity, adventure, or challenge that you've been interested in. Maybe acne won't let you feel the satisfaction of doing something that displays your talents or lets you feel proud of yourself. Acne likes to look at you and say, "You think *this* is yours to enjoy, but it's not." *This* could be anything, whatever it is that brings the feeling of value and purpose to your life. When you look closely at rules and restrictions in your life, it could be that you've been inadvertently labeling what is good for you as "bad" as a result of acne's degrading and self-defeating messages.

Starting now, it's important to stop believing what acne says. It's a stupid zit, nothing more. If acne's main premise about you is false—that you're not allowed to live your life because you'd be "bad" if you did—then the logic behind its rules and regulations is false too. Acne is just an immature bully that's trying to create a mind block for you, built out of dead ends that pop up every time you want to move forward in your life. These dead ends aren't real, they're just enforced using fear, superstition, and punishment. Because they're not real, you can venture forward past them and see that the road does continue.

Having acne on your face doesn't mean that you should restrict your life more than what acne's already trying to do. It means that it's time to stand up for what you want and leave acne behind in your rearview mirror.

Sometimes, you just have to break your own rules. It may seem counterintuitive, but when you let yourself be bad at times, you can end up feeling healthier and more balanced in your life than if you're always trying to be good. The rules we construct around acne don't always make sense, and they can actually block our way toward better skin as we've talked about. If breaking the rules makes you feel "bad," enjoy the feeling for what it is. Most likely, you need a healthy dose of bad in order to strengthen your boundaries against acne and make it less of a priority in your life.

We can look to kids for inspiration on how to break rules, because kids are naturally experts on doing this. If a rule seems bendable to them and they want to test it, they'll disobey and see what happens next. Of course it's preferable to have limits around how far kids go with this, but in healthy doses, it's great for kids to break rules from time to time. It allows them to explore, learn, have fun, and get to know themselves out in the world. Acne tries to take this type of joy and learning away from us. It demands that we enter a no man's land where we can't be a kid any longer, but we also can't enter adulthood and trust in our own decisions. The result can be maddening, and it can often make you feel like nothing is allowed, period.

No more asking permission from this bully, and for that matter, no more asking permission from *any* bully. Being "bad" and breaking the rules in healthy doses is a right that you have, and acne doesn't have the right to take it away from you. Acne will continue to label what you do as either good and obedient, or bad and disobedient. No matter what it says, you can find relief for your skin when you practice ignoring acne's rude voice. As you get in tune with your adventurous spirit and stray away from overly restrictive rules, you can diffuse the fears that acne has constructed around your life. You can enjoy more of what you do, and worry less about what you "shouldn't do." Acne's fear-based mentality is what it uses to invade your skin, so in leaving that mindset behind you'll find that over time acne has less power over your skin and your life. Why miss out on potentially good things in your life just because acne's mislabeling them as bad?

CHAPTER 17

Back in Your Own Skin

———————————•—————————

These days, it's common to feel like doing things for yourself or spending time on your own are guilty pleasures. If you do things for someone else, that's totally fine, but the minute you direct energy toward yourself, the mind can signal alarm bells as if something's wrong. "I should be doing stuff for someone else, or attending to my to-do list," the mind says. "I should be doing anything but enjoying my own company." We hear a lot about the importance of community from everywhere, and the types of benefits a social network offers. While having supportive people around you is great, we don't hear much about how important it is to have time and space for yourself. Standing up to acne and getting back in your own skin means learning how to be comfortable on your own too, and allowing yourself to *enjoy who you are.*

Those of us who deal with acne will also often grapple with a heightened feeling that it's important to make everyone else happy, often at the exclusion of ourselves. We may be extreme in believing that life is about pleasing others, and we may drain our own energy by giving it to other people and withholding it from ourselves. By acne's very mindset, it encourages extreme self-sacrifice. It says: Don't be seen. Be small. Don't shine. Believe what others say about you. Give away everything you have. Over time, this skin condition that mainstream medicine describes as "just physical" can become a belief system. The belief is built around you being the least important person in your life, while everyone else—including the bully acne—becomes the priority. We end up leaving ourselves behind.

In addition, there are too many outside influences these days that try and take us away from ourselves. Internet, media, politics, entertainment, social spheres, and sometimes even the guy waiting at the street corner for the bus seem to all have opinions on what is the best way to live. The best way that people say to live hardly ever involves you being there for yourself first, it more often involves mindlessly following or doing whatever they're saying or doing. Modern life can get incredibly overwhelming at times and, of course, frequently lead to breakouts for those dealing with acne. The place you can go to feel grounded when everything around you seems haywire, chaotic, confusing, or stressful is:

Back in your own skin.

We're told the opposite message by acne, and by the mainstream health and skin care industries. When life is stressful, we're encouraged to distrust our skin because acne resides there, and because we supposedly don't know how to cultivate clarity for our skin or our lives. We're instantly judged by the label of this four-letter word, and rather than feeling like we have innate potential for health in our skin already, we come to believe that we have to run far away from who we are in order to be perfect some day. On top of that, we're urged to attack our skin with harsh products and medicines that further disrupt its integrity. If our skin starts screaming back in protest and displaying even worse breakouts of acne, it's actually because it's trying to be there for us and we're not letting it.

The groundedness and comfort we can return to inside ourselves, especially during tough times, is our first home. We can walk anywhere on this planet, and no matter what happens we have the benefit of being able to reside in our own skin at the same time. We're like turtles in a way, and the protective layer we possess is the skin instead of a shell. Our protective cover is a lot tougher and more adaptable than we give it credit for. In the busy rat race of a life we sometimes get entrenched in, the comfort of our first home can often feel out of reach. We may feel influence from all around us to leave this home behind in order to better connect with the world and with other people. The truth is actually the opposite: The more at home we feel in our own skin, the better adapted we'll be to getting through challenges in the world and interacting with others—and the less that acne and other bullying influences can invade our skin. Sure, they may try. But we're at home and providing natural strength to the skin through our spirit and the courage to be with ourselves.

Don't forget about you. Your skin loves it when you spend time with yourself, in other words finding opportunities for "me time." When you step away from it all and honor your existence by hanging out with yourself, the skin is rejuvenated in a way that may not be immediately visible on the surface, but can shine through over the long-term. Living in your skin means allowing yourself to do what *you* want, not always jumping to what you imagine others want from you.

One way you could use your time is to relax and unwind, taking a break from the worries and anxieties that can accumulate during day-to-day life. Today, a ton of emphasis is put on being social all the time, but many of us need healthy breaks from the social aspects of life in order to reconnect with ourselves and our own skin. As we've talked about, not all social influences are healthy for us, and it can be helpful to step back from stressful environments at times to reflect on what we need for ourselves. Without knowing it, we may be spending more time on getting lost in the social world or in satisfying other people's needs than is healthy for us. Taking a break from people is often the best way to reconnect with taking care of yourself too.

Other times, life gets so busy and full to the point where it feels like our obligations are dragging us around and we're just watching life go by. Today's world tends to put a lot of pressure on us to be on top of things and striving for success all the time. Even though it may be tough to mentally take a breather while your to-do list is unchecked, you'll thank yourself afterward when your stress levels go down and you have more energy for yourself. Try and think about which elements of your life feel controlling to the point of fatigue or exhaustion, and allow yourself to rest and take back the reins. Just like we don't want acne dictating our lives, we also don't want other external circumstances to take over daily life, drain our energy, and stress out our skin—as much as we can help it.

Getting back in your skin can also involve reconnecting with a hobby, skill, or activity you enjoy putting your energy toward. Maybe you're a writer who abandoned writing a novel halfway through, and now it's time to get back to it. You could be someone who loves playing music, and it's been too long since you've exercised your musical chops. You may enjoy cooking, drawing, playing a sport, teaching, or hiking, and you've just been waiting to return to it at some point. It doesn't have to be gung-ho, but you can start doing what is fun for you again if it's been a while. Again, it may not be obvious why doing something you enjoy is good for your skin. Living comfortably in your skin starts with your life first, and when you're engaged in what makes you excited, curious, and energized, your skin will feel the effects both inside and out.

As far as being social, there's someone who has potentially been waiting the longest to hang out with you—*you*. Your own company is where real connection can spark in your life, even before you start branching out and interacting with other people. When you value your presence, you can start to hear your own voice again and it will often times help allay worries and doubts that have felt overwhelming. Worries and doubts will surface at times throughout life, whether about acne or anything else, but we have a friend in ourselves that we can turn to unconditionally for support. We first need to see ourselves as an important ally in our own lives. Acne tries to thwart this natural friendship every chance it gets, but when we take a step back to return to our own skin and listen to ourselves, acne's message instantly starts to weaken and continues to do so.

Step nineteen in facing acne: Hang out with yourself and reconnect with your own voice.

The more comfortable you get in your skin, you may find that your skin is less reactive and irritable over time. It has become used to living with acne as a constant companion, and in this bully's presence, it doesn't get much of a chance to enjoy its natural strength and integrity. The four-letter word encourages it to feel deflated, lackluster, and frustrated instead. When you reconnect with yourself, you help give real confidence back to your skin. As a result, your skin isn't as fazed by acne's stupid and cowardly behavior. You're giving it the very nourishment and courage it needs, just by being there for yourself more. Acne will gradually feel outnumbered, as you and your skin team up and stop taking its crap.

Conversely, the less you live in your skin, the more that acne and other people can get under it. "Getting under my skin" is a common expression people use to express when someone has upset them and it's hard to stop thinking about it. This is exactly acne's aim, as well as the aim of other bullying influences that may try and mess with you. If you're being honest, you know deep down that you don't want influences like this making their home under your skin. If that's the case, don't let anyone displace you from the home that's yours and yours alone. It's a place that you're welcome in anytime, and from there you'll find the strength you need to face acne and any other challenges.

CHAPTER 18
Acne's Just Not Worth It

———— • ————

You may be sitting here right now having already invested a lot of time, money, energy, and thought on acne. The mission to defeat this four-letter word has probably felt exhausting on a daily basis and oftentimes become an obstacle to other things you want to do in life. At the same time, it has a lot of momentum behind it. When you've already dedicated so much of yourself to this fight, it may seem like a deflating idea to abandon this arena and try something else. Even if you haven't had positive results from your efforts, it can still be hard to give up on something you spent so much on, especially if everyone else from doctors to family members seem to suggest it's the best way to go. They say to keep hunting for the acne solution and to fight your skin into submission until acne goes away. But something's missing here, and we all know it the longer we keep fighting the same fight.

What's missing? It's the honest truth that a small zit is attempting to control our lives with its disrespect, pompousness, and profane messages. What seems like a fight against acne actually plays right into its hands and allows it to mistreat us further. We rearrange our lives around for acne, ask for its permission before making decisions, and assume a lot of blame and guilt when our skin breaks out. As we bow down to this little word and roll out a red carpet for it, it gains more control over us and treats us worse. The fight isn't helping, and it's being directed at the wrong side: We end up fighting ourselves and our skin more than acne itself.

Acne wants us to get embroiled with it in an endless and heated battle and to hurt ourselves in the process. It wants us to direct anger inward and to attack our skin. It wants us to give up on our appearance and hand it over. It wants us to see ourselves in the worst light and to accept the branding of ACNE for life. This bully's never going to change its puny and narrow mindset, but we can change by quitting its stupid and wasteful fight. It's not a fair fight and it never has been—the odds are always stacked in acne's favor as it makes sure the rules are rigged against us.

Don't fight your skin and yourself. That's just giving acne what it wants.

Stand up to acne instead, not by going to war with it, but by showing it that it's not the focus of your life. Acne's not worth your energy: It's not worth listening to, thinking about, or structuring your life around. *It's not worth fighting.* Acne, and other bullies like it, crave a lot of attention from any individual who is just living his or her own life. Every day you're supposed to work for acne, lowering yourself and placing this little pimple on a pedestal where it sits and barks out orders. Eventually, you just get sick of it. It's not a rewarding job and the efforts you make don't get you anywhere, other than farther away from your own life. There comes a time when you want the spotlight back on you and off acne, and that takes remembering that you're different from this four-letter word.

Acne competes with you for attention on a daily basis, but there's no real competition there. It's like comparing apples and oranges. Even though acne implies you're both the same, its messages are pure trickery and intended to make you and your skin more vulnerable to its trespassing. You're completely separate from acne, with your own identity and your own voice that can overcome acne as you stop taking this bully seriously. Is acne a serious issue? As a society, we tend to make it more serious than it needs to be, almost deferring to it like some sort of authority figure. This is fake authority that's not to be trusted.

When you boil it down, acne is just using its bratty behavior to try and order you around, and there's no wisdom or authority in that. Whether it's acne or a brat you encounter out in the world who tries to trigger stress and disorder in your life, you don't owe these bullying influences anything, let alone your obedience. Don't bother trying to please them or make them happy and satisfied, because that's exactly what they want. It gets you more involved in the struggle they create for you. Pay as little attention to them as possible, and you'll start your journey toward putting them last and putting yourself (and your skin) first.

The more you can recognize that acne has a big social component to it, the more you'll have protection from it in the long-term. It's common for people to break out worse after interacting with family members or friends who are in the habit of treating them disrespectfully and like a child. You can't just blame the severity of the breakout on the nebulous idea of "stress." This is a specific kind of stress that's coming from an unhealthy dynamic—that of someone who is trying to bring you down using their words, actions, and controlling behavior. Bullying individuals or groups who are in your life undermine the health of your skin the longer they belittle you, and the only person who can establish a boundary to this mistreatment is you.

Likewise, any messages coming from society, the media, or mainstream culture that suggest you're "wrong" as you are and that you need to prove yourself to everyone else are not worth listening to. The purpose of life isn't to prove yourself to those who seek to hold you back and mislabel you. It's just as important to establish a boundary against these disparaging voices, because they don't know who you are and they're wrong. You have richness in your own life that is already present, and this value can be harder to appreciate when you're prioritizing what others say, including acne. Whether it's coming from acne, the small sphere of people you know, or the world at large, messages that tell you to place ideals and blind conformity ahead of yourself can become a threat to your own skin.

As you keep your eyes open to how these messages may be affecting your skin's health, you can practice rejecting them and showing them that they're not invited into your life anymore. When it comes to long-standing dynamics with other people and social environments, you can't expect an overnight change. Life's also not perfect, so you'll still find yourself dealing with people who don't respect your boundaries and aren't willing to change moving forward. However, the longer you keep building your boundaries, the better you get at pushing these influences out of the way as much as possible and taking care of yourself. As you do, you create space for healthier additions to your life. That can be anything you want, including clearer skin over time.

Regardless of the immediate results, these habits support the underlying integrity of your skin and its natural defense against acne. You can start to enjoy what's uniquely yours, including your appearance, with less guilt about it. It becomes easier to recognize that your skin is on your side and not against you, and you two can work together rather than fight each other. You get to reconnect with yourself, and appreciate what you have going for you. These changes can help spark long-lasting strength and protection for your skin more than any skin care line, supplement, pharmaceutical, or other "quick fix" can do for you.

Inside almost every person who deals with acne is a voice that screams out, "Why do I have to do all this stuff just to have clear skin?!" Good question, and you can investigate the answer to it. The effort toward getting better skin can feel like a penance, as if you've brought acne on yourself. This four-letter word is blaming you for everything and giving you attitude on a daily basis. What are you going to do about it? Acne's just not worth your attention, and you can weaken its "power" by ignoring it and moving on with your life. We are dealing with four little letters that are getting blown way out of proportion, and because of this heightened focus on acne, we may unintentionally be inviting it to stick around longer.

It's time to kick this unwelcome guest out of your house, and regardless of what anyone else says, you can do it. The story is still being written for your skin, and what you're seeing right now while battling acne is not the final outcome. I repeat, it's not the ending, and quite possibly it's the beginning of a new story where you can make a real difference for not only the clarity of your skin but also your life. You can reconnect with what you *want to* invite into your life, and you can help write the story rather than letting these four letters dictate what it should be. Take a chance: Try and work on your mindset surrounding acne and see what effects the change in thinking has on your skin. Always remember, acne is just another four-letter word.

If you experience improvement in your skin going forward and acne re-enters the picture occasionally, keep your determination to enforce a boundary against it. It's common for people to see clear evidence of their skin improving, only to find it backsliding again after some time. If this happens to you too, that's okay, it doesn't mean that you've lost progress with your skin. There are just ups and downs to this experience, as well as plateaus where you may not get results as quickly as you want. You just have to be patient.

The goal isn't to find the perfect solution to acne, like so many people are selling out there in the form of gimmicks and fads. That approach just doesn't work, whether it's sold in a bottle or as a way of thinking. You don't need a perfect solution or a perfect life to enjoy clear skin. Living your life, your way, is what will allow your clear skin to shine through.

There will always be bullies like acne and disrespectful people out there, they don't simply disappear. But we don't have to listen to what they say about us, and we can live our lives in spite of them. Find strength in your real voice, the one that tells you the truth about who you are no matter how many curse words acne screams out.

Some people may feel anxious about their skin improving as they notice others admiring it. This may be hard to believe, because you'd expect that the most anxiety would come from having noticeable acne. Still, it can be quite a change to see people looking at you and your skin differently, and it's normal if some nerves are triggered from this new experience. When your skin is feeling good, enjoy it and you'll get more adapted to the improvement over time.

Finally, keep your eyes ahead as much as possible toward your own experience of standing up to acne. Everyone's journey with their skin is unique, and you can't accurately compare what you're going through with other people's results. Whether your skin seems "better" or "worse" compared to someone else's skin doesn't matter, and it doesn't give you real clues toward how you can have the skin you want. As you're ignoring acne, try and ignore comparisons to other people as well.

One last thing to keep in mind. The suggestions in this book can help with other health complaints you may be experiencing too. Are you dealing with digestive upset, hormone imbalance, weight gain, trouble sleeping, anxiety, a skin condition, or other difficult-to-treat symptom? Most chronic health issues, while treated as purely physical by the medical system, have mental, emotional, and social roots to them just like acne does. When you stand up for who you are and define your boundaries, as we've talked about, you clear the path for your whole body to experience better energy, health, and vitality.

Next, we'll recap a list of twelve simple tools for standing up to acne. You might want to keep these tips handy on your mirror or refrigerator so that if you start fixating on acne and getting too involved in its drama, you can return to the list and get back on track.

In the final chapter, we'll talk about one way that you can write an opening to the next part of your skin's story. It doesn't matter if you do the writing in your head or on paper, but you may find that the act of expressing what you have to say sparks your desire to be rid of acne in a brand new way. As we near the end of this book, I'd like to share with you one take-home message from everything we've talked about so far:

Don't let acne stop you from living your life, because this four-letter word isn't worth it.

CHAPTER 19
Twelve Tools for Standing Up to Acne

1. Pay as little attention to acne as possible—and walk away from the mirror if you're staring at it for too long.
2. Recognize the profane words and messages that this four-letter word is using against you.
3. Question acne's authority to police your skin and your life.
4. Be a friend to yourself and listen to your unique voice (that is separate from acne's voice).
5. Learn to accept your flaws and challenges, and set your own bar rather than trying to live up to acne's or other people's expectations of you.
6. Catch acne red-handed when it's planting fears and superstitions in your head.
7. Head out of the room you're tempted to hide in, and see what happens next.
8. Give yourself a healthy dose of "bad" from time to time.
9. If you're mad at acne and influences like it, it's okay to admit that.
10. Don't wait for a miracle, and take steps forward that *make sense* to you.
11. Treat yourself how you want to be treated, and then you can learn where to place boundaries with others.
12. Say bye to acne starting now, and live your life.

CHAPTER 20

So Long, Sucker

—————•—————

Writing a goodbye letter to acne is one way that you can start saying bye to acne right now, by asserting that you're separate from it and ready to leave it behind. More than simply being symbolic, the act of putting your thoughts down on paper helps you to begin the process of letting go of this long-standing bully, and it prepares you for upcoming changes to your life from making this decision. You're also getting a chance to tell acne off, because after all, it's been cursing at you for a long time. Now you get to speak your mind. With this statement you're off the hook and you don't have to work for acne or be tested by it anymore.

Your letter doesn't have to be long, and you can repeat this act whenever you're feeling doubts about getting rid of acne. Like everything we've talked about in this book, the letter is not meant to be a quick fix for what you've been going through. However, the more you reconnect with yourself and what you want, the stronger the platform you build for standing up to acne. You start planting seeds that can help support clearer skin over the long-term, and you never know when they'll sprout.

Below is just an example, and I encourage you to write one in your own words too. Go ahead and say whatever you have to say to acne's four little letters. At this point, I wish you the best and leave you to write, type, or think about your letter and the next chapter of your skin's journey.

Yo Acne,

Just writing to let you know that you don't matter to me. I'm tired of fighting you or trying to appease you, and I have other things I want to do with my time and energy moving forward. Don't expect me to pay attention to you like I have been, because my eyes are open to what you're doing and I don't respect it. I choose to live without your drama. I also don't respect anyone who treats me like you do. My skin is my home and you can all get lost.

You don't know me and what you're saying about me is just plain wrong. You and I are not the same, and I'm not obligated to you. Go ahead and waste your time trying to mess with me if you want, but you're a coward who's no match for me at the end of the day. You're just another four-letter word and you can't stop me from living my life.

So long sucker.

ACKNOWLEDGMENTS

First I'd like to thank my multitalented editor, Jason Petersen, who just got it when it came to editing this book. His insight, patience, and creative eye helped me push on through finishing it, even when I couldn't see the horizon. I couldn't ask for a better editor.

Thank you also to my patients who have come in over the years to ask for help with acne and other skin conditions. You trusted me to deliver something different, and what I learned help me bring this book to life.

I appreciate the talented work of Will Silva, who made the interior of my book bold and eye-catching. You can find his quality formatting services at www.fiverr.com/tlmason.

For the cover design, a big shout-out to Bojan and his team at Pixelstudio. Consistently, they have been creating beautiful covers for my books. You can find their services at www.fiverr.com/pixelstudio.

ABOUT THE AUTHOR

A arti Patel is a naturopathic doctor and author who enjoys writing about health, as well as fiction that explores individuality and society's impact on health. She lives in the Pacific Northwest with her family and finds rainy days to be perfect for writing and watching movie marathons. She believes that health is not about perfect diets, hours spent at the gym, a magic cure from supplements or pharmaceuticals, or any one particular belief or ideology. Rather, it's life itself, how we treat it and support it, and the courageous actions of the individual in the face of real life challenges.

To learn about her other titles, please visit www.d2books.com.

TO THE
READER

———————— • ————————

Thank you for taking the time to read my book! It means a lot that you would choose my work out of the many acne books that are available. I hope you found something in here that uniquely relates to your experience and helps your skin.

I always appreciate honest reviews on Amazon by anyone who has something to share about reading or using the book. So many people are struggling with acne, and your opinion of what you read here may be valuable to someone.

I wish you the best as you head out into the world and reclaim what's yours from acne.

www.ingramcontent.com/pod-product-compliance
Lightning Source LLC
Chambersburg PA
CBHW022112280326
41933CB00007B/356